Clinical Decisions in Medically Complex Dental Patients, Part I

Editors

MEL MUPPARAPU
ANDRES PINTO

DENTAL CLINICS OF NORTH AMERICA

www.dental.theclinics.com

July 2023 • Volume 67 • Number 3

ELSEVIER

1600 John F. Kennedy Boulevard • Suite 1800 • Philadelphia, Pennsylvania, 19103-2899

http://www.dental.theclinics.com

DENTAL CLINICS OF NORTH AMERICA Volume 67, Number 3
July 2023 ISSN 0011-8532, ISBN: 978-0-323-93921-8

Editor: John Vassallo; j.vassallo@elsevier.com
Developmental Editor: Akshay Samson

Dental Clinics of North America (ISSN 0011-8532) is published quarterly by Elsevier Inc., 360 Park Avenue South, New York, NY 10010-1710. Months of issue are January, April, July, and October. Business and Editorial Offices: 1600 John F. Kennedy Boulevard, Suite 1800, Philadelphia, PA 19103-2899. Periodicals postage paid at New York, NY and additional mailing offices. Subscription prices are $333.00 per year (domestic individuals), $692.00 per year (domestic institutions), $100.00 per year (domestic students/residents), $388.00 per year (Canadian individuals), $897.00 per year (Canadian institutions), $100.00 per year (Canadian students/residents) $454.00 per year (international individuals), $897.00 per year (international institutions), and $200.00 per year (international students/residents). International air speed delivery is included in all *Clinics* subscription prices. All prices are subject to change without notice. **POSTMASTER:** Send address changes to *Dental Clinics of North America*, Elsevier Health Sciences Division, Subscription Customer Service, 3251 Riverport Lane, Maryland Heights, MO 63043. **Customer Service (orders, claims, online, change of address): Elsevier Health Sciences Division, Subscription Customer Service, 3251 Riverport Lane, Maryland Heights, MO 63043. Tel: 1-800-654-2452 (U.S. and Canada). Fax: 314-447-8029. E-mail: journalscustomerservice-usa@elsevier.com (for print support); journalsonlinesupport-usa@elsevier. com (for online support).**

Reprints. For copies of 100 or more, of articles in this publication, please contact the Commercial Reprints Department, Elsevier Inc., 360 Park Avenue South, New York, NY 10010-1710. Tel.: 212-633-3874; Fax: 212-633-3820; E-mail: reprints@elsevier.com.

The *Dental Clinics of North America* is covered in *MEDLINE/PubMed (Index Medicus), Current Contents/Clinical Medicine, ISI/BIOMED* and *Clinahl*.

Contributors

EDITORS

MEL MUPPARAPU, DMD, MDS
Diplomate, American Board of Oral and Maxillofacial Radiology; Director, Oral and Maxillofacial Radiology, Professor of Clinical Oral Medicine, Department of Oral Medicine, University of Pennsylvania School of Dental Medicine, Philadelphia, Pennsylvania, USA

ANDRES PINTO, DMD, MPH, MBA, MSCE
Diplomate, American Board of Oral Medicine; Chair and Professor, Oral and Maxillofacial Medicine and Diagnostic Sciences, Case Western Reserve University School of Dental Medicine, Cleveland, Ohio, USA

AUTHORS

ENITAN ADEGITE, MD, MPH
Associate Professor of Pediatrics, Drexel University, St Christopher's Children Hospital, Philadelphia, Pennsylvania, USA

FATMAH ALHENDI, BMedSc, DDS, MSOB
Alqurain, Kuwait; Ministry of health, Jaber AlAhmad Dental Specialty Center, South Surra, Ministries Zone, Kuwait

ANWAR A. ALMUZAINI, BMedSc, BDM, MSOB
Ministry of Health, Jaber AlAhmad Dental Specialty Center, South Surra, Ministries Zone, Kuwait

DALAL ALOMAR, DDS, MS
Oral Medicine Specialist, Ministry of Health, Jaber AlAhmad Dental Specialty Center, South Surra, Ministries Zone, Kuwait

PAULA L. COATES, DDS, MS
Pediatric Dentistry, Children's Hospital of Richmond, Richmond, Virginia, USA

ANDRES DAVILA, DMD
Department of Oral Medicine, University of Pennsylvania School of Dental Medicine, Philadelphia, Pennsylvania, USA

ADEYINKA DAYO, BDS, DMD, MS
Assistant Professor, Department of Oral Medicine, University of Pennsylvania School of Dental Medicine, Philadelphia, Pennsylvania, USA

KATHERINE FRANCE, DMD, MBE
Assistant Professor, Department of Oral Medicine, University of Pennsylvania School of Dental Medicine, Philadelphia, Pennsylvania, USA

KAROLINE E. GENUNG, RDH, BS, PHDHP
Public Health Dental Hygiene Practioner, Division of Community Oral Health, University of Pennsylvania School of Dental Medicine, Philadelphia, Pennsylvania, USA

CHIZOBAM IDAHOSA, BDS, DDS, MS
Clinical Associate Professor, Department of Oral Medicine, University of Pennsylvania School of Dental Medicine, Philadelphia, Pennsylvania, USA

OSAMUDIAMEN IDAHOSA, MD, FCCP
Attending Physician, Department of Critical Care Medicine, St Luke's University Health Network, Bethlehem, Pennsylvania, USA

JAYAKUMAR JAYARAMAN, BDS, MDS, FDSRCS, MS, PhD
Pediatric Dentistry, Children's Hospital of Richmond, Richmond, Virginia, USA

LEONARD JENSEN, DMD
Assistant Professor, Clinical Director, Division of Community Oral Health, University of Pennsylvania School of Dental Medicine, Philadelphia, Pennsylvania, USA

KENNETH KUFTA, DMD, MD
Oral and Maxillofacial Surgeon, Hospital of the University of Pennsylvania, Philadelphia, Pennsylvania, USA

PAYAM MIRFENDERESKI, DDS
Chief Resident, Department of Oral Medicine, University of Pennsylvania School of Dental Medicine, Philadelphia, Pennsylvania, USA

NIKHIL MISTRY, DMD, MD
Oral and Maxillofacial Surgeon, Hospital of the University of Pennsylvania, Philadelphia, Pennsylvania, USA

MEL MUPPARAPU, DMD, MDS
Diplomate, American Board of Oral and Maxillofacial Radiology; Director, Oral and Maxillofacial Radiology, Professor of Clinical Oral Medicine, Department of Oral Medicine, University of Pennsylvania School of Dental Medicine, Philadelphia, Pennsylvania, USA

SCOTT ODELL, DMD
Associate Professor, Division of Community Oral Health, University of Pennsylvania School of Dental Medicine, Philadelphia, Pennsylvania, USA

TEMITOPE T. OMOLEHINWA, BDS, DMD, DScD
Assistant Professor, Department of Oral Medicine, Penn Dental Medicine University of Pennsylvania, Philadelphia, Pennsylvania, USA

NEERAJ PANCHAL, DMD, MD, MA
Assistant Professor of Oral and Maxillofacial Surgery and Pharmacology, Penn Dental Medicine, Section Chief of Oral and Maxillofacial Surgery, Penn Presbyterian Medical Center, Philadelphia VA Hospitals, Philadelphia, Pennsylvania, USA

ANDRES PINTO, DMD, MPH, MBA, MSCE
Diplomate, American Board of Oral Medicine; Chair and Professor, Oral and Maxillofacial Medicine and Diagnostic Sciences, Case Western Reserve University School of Dental Medicine, Cleveland, Ohio, USA

JILLIAN RIGERT, DMD, MD
Postdoctoral Research Fellow, Department of Radiation Oncology, The University of Texas MD Anderson Cancer Center, Houston, Texas, USA

MIRIAM R. ROBBINS, DDS, MS
Department of Oral Medicine, Director, Care Center for Persons with Disabilities, Professor of Clinical Oral Medicine and Clinical Restorative Dentistry, The University of Pennsylvania School of Dental Medicine, Philadelphia, Pennsylvania, USA

KIMBERLY A. STRAUCH, PhD, CRNP, ANP-BC
Executive Director, Leonard A. Lauder Community Care Nurse Practitioner Program, Department of Oral Medicine, Care Center for Persons with Disabilities, The University of Pennsylvania School of Dental Medicine, The University of Pennsylvania School of Nursing, Philadelphia, Pennsylvania, USA

ALI Z. SYED, BDS, MHA, MS
Diplomate, American Board of Oral and Maxillofacial Radiology; Assistant Professor, Oral and Maxillofacial Medicine and Diagnostic Services, Case Western University School of Dental Medicine, Cleveland, Ohio, USA

Contents

Patients with cooccurring coronary artery disease and arrhythmias are frequently encountered by dental providers. Individuals with comorbid cardiovascular disease who require dual anticoagulant and antiplatelet therapy are a clinical challenge with regard to the need to balance the risks and benefits of intensive antithrombotic therapy. Modifications to dental care will need to be individualized considering the current disease state and medical management. Oral health promotion and good oral hygiene measures are recommended among this population.

Heart failure (HF) and valve replacements are common conditions encountered by dental professionals. Identification and differentiation between acute versus chronic HF symptoms will be key to providing safe and effective dental care. Vasoactive agents should be used cautiously in individuals with advanced HF. People with underlying cardiac conditions that put them at an increased risk of developing infectious endocarditis require antibiotic prophylaxis before all dental procedures. Establishing and maintaining optimal oral health is necessary to minimize the risks of bacterial seeding from the oral cavity to the heart.

Management of the diabetic dental patient should focus on the delivery of comprehensive dental care with an emphasis on maintaining periodontal health. Gingivitis, periodontitis, and associated bone loss independent of plaque accumulation are associated with poorly controlled diabetes. Periodontal status should be monitored carefully in patients with diabetes and underlying disease managed aggressively. Likewise, the dental team plays an important role in the identification of hypertension and managing dental-related side effects of anti-hypertensives.

controlled asthma and modify dental treatment accordingly. Prevention of an acute asthma exacerbation is key. Patients should be reminded to bring their rescue inhaler with them to every dental appointment. Patients who are using inhaled corticosteroids to manage their asthma are at greater risk of oral candidiasis, xerostomia, and caries. Regular dental visits and good oral hygiene are important among this population.

Cardiovascular diseases are among the most common medical problems in the general population. Individuals with underlying cardiac conditions require special considerations with regard to appropriateness of dental treatment and precautions needed to deliver safe and effective care. Patients with unstable cardiac disease are at higher risk of developing complications during dental treatment. Similarly, comorbid conditions among patients with ischemic heart disease, such as chronic obstructive pulmonary disease, can further affect dental health and treatment, and they often require more individualized dental approaches.

As public health stewards, dental providers must be mindful of actual of potential infectious disease risks. Tuberculosis (TB) is a leading cause of death in adults worldwide and is spread via aerosolized droplets. Individuals at the greatest risk of contracting TB are those with impaired immunity or those who have a higher risk of being exposed to an infection due to environmental factors. Dental providers must be aware of the clinical and public health implications of treating people with active versus latent TB infections.

Early dental screening and treatment before and after solid organ transplantation are recommended infection prophylaxis measures. Dental treatment after transplantation should only be rendered after a discussion with the patient's health-care provider and/or transplant surgeon to determine the patient's stability for dental care. Potential sources of acute or chronic oral infections should be evaluated at every visit. Periodontal evaluation and through dental prophylaxis should be performed. Oral hygiene instruction including the importance of maintaining excellent oral health after transplant should be reviewed.

A 13-year old male patient with uncontrolled asthma presents with a grossly decayed permanent first molar. Medical consultation was obtained

Mönckeberg medial arteriosclerosis is a condition characterized by the calcification of the tunica media layer of the blood vessels that are visible on plain radiography or sectional tomography. In dentistry, a properly acquired panoramic radiograph may show the condition incidentally. It is also known as medial arterial calcinosis and can be associated with diabetes mellitus or chronic kidney disease. This condition is different from the more common atherosclerosis where the tunica intima remains unaffected, and the diameter of the vessel lumen is preserved. Dental treatment can be performed when the patient is stable with medically controlled diabetes.

The authors describe the management of a 57-year-old man with hemophilia A who presents for extractions and implant placements. The patient required a combination of extractions, scaling and root planning, and composite restorations. The authors describe the management protocol for this patient as well as general considerations in the management of patients with hemophilia A.

Von Willebrand disease is a platelet phase bleeding disorder, affecting platelet aggregation and adhesion. It can be inherited or acquired in origin. Patients with von Willebrand disease can be successfully treated in a dental setting. This article discusses the dental management of a 74-year-old white woman presenting with pain and gingival erythema in the maxillary anterior area. The article emphasizes the importance of consultation with the hematologist in treating patients with von Willebrand disease, and understanding that disease severity varies in patients. A patient-specific protocol recommended by the hematologist should be followed for each patient.

A 7-year-old girl came to the Emergency Department following an avulsion of the maxillary central incisor. The tooth was replanted and splinted. The patient was referred to a hematologist for follow-up and maintenance of adequate levels of Factor VIII.

Intraosseous arteriovenous malformations in jaws are rare congenital vascular abnormalities that the dentist may encounter. A vascular lesion or disease should be suspected when there is unexplained bleeding from the oral cavity. Diagnostic imaging is a valuable tool in diagnosing and localizing vascular lesions. An understanding of some of the salient clinical and radiographic features of arteriovenous malformations in jaws aids the clinician in correctly diagnosing this condition and avoids iatrogenic injuries, such as hasty tooth extraction, which may potentially cause severe bleeding and possibly death. The dentist should acknowledge their expertise/limitation, and know when the need for referral arises.

A 26-year-old man living with HIV and depression presents with symptoms of tooth sensitivity. His laboratory studies are all within normal limits except for a high viral load. The patient does not require any special dental management protocol and should be treated like other patients, with his laboratory studies reviewed every 6 months to 1 year. HIV is now a chronic medical conditions, with most patients having stable disease if they are compliant with their medications. Universal infection control protocols should be followed for all patients regardless of their HIV status.

A 34-year-old male patient living with human immunodeficiency virus (HIV) presents to the dental clinic with a 1-week history of throbbing tooth pain. He was referred by an oral medicine specialist for evaluation and treatment. The patient presents with very low absolute neutrophil, platelet, and cluster of differentiation (CD) (also T-helper cell) 4+ cell counts, as well as a high HIV RNA/viral load. Determining factors for dental management before extraction of the offending teeth were the absolute neutrophil count and platelet counts.

A 50-year-old female patient with a history of HIV, uncontrolled diabetes, hyperlipidemia, hypertension, and chronic hepatitis C presents for dental evaluation and treatment because of bleeding gums. This article discusses modifications to her dental management with respect to her various medical conditions. Noninfectious comorbid conditions especially diabetes, cardiovascular disease, and hyperlipidemia are common findings in patients with HIV. Modifications to dental treatment should not be based solely on HIV RNA (viral load) and $CD4^+$ cell count. Dentists can play a role in ensuring patients' comorbid medical conditions are well managed.

seizure is suspected and other causes of altered consciousness or involuntary motor movements are ruled out, proper management should commence immediately. The first step in management is to immediately remove/stop all provocative factors, like bright flashing lights, drill sounds, and such. Benzodiazepines remain as the first-line treatment for patients with continued seizures before activating emergency medical services.

Accidental foreign body aspiration is not uncommon during a dental procedure and remains a real risk for many dental procedures. Although approximately 50% of patients are asymptomatic after aspiration of a foreign body, understanding the appropriate next steps in management of these patients is critical in preventing morbid and even lethal outcomes in some instances. Appropriate knowledge of identification and management of such instances is important for all practicing dentists. This article goes into the diagnosis and management of both uncomplicated foreign body ingestion and complicated foreign body aspirations.

Although dental treatment in a patient with well-controlled type 2 diabetes mellitus is uncomplicated, hypoglycemia is one of the most dreaded complications among diabetics and remains as one of the leading causes of endocrine medical emergencies. Identification and prompt treatment is important to all dental practitioners. This scenario goes into the diagnosis and management of medication-induced hypoglycemia.

Dentists should be trained to treat any allergic reaction in a dental office, and in this scenario, allergic reaction to latex-based product (rubber dam) is illustrated. Identification of signs and symptoms related to latex allergies is vital, and all dentists should be trained in the appropriate management of such a patient. The dental management of the scenario describes details of the diagnosis and management of latex-related allergies in a dental office for both adults and children.

Dentists should be equipped to treat any allergic reaction in a dental office and in this scenario, anaphylaxis is noted after administration of a penicillin derivative given before a dental procedure. Identification of signs and symptoms related to anaphylaxis is vital and appropriate management of the patient is the key. The dental management of the scenario goes into the diagnosis and management of anaphylaxis in a dental office.

including the stage and level of control. Patients on hemodialysis are ideally seen the day after dialysis with consideration to arteriovenous shunt placement for blood pressure measurement and avoiding or changing the dose of certain drugs based on the patient's glomerular filtration rate. Drugs cleared during hemodialysis may require a supplemental dose. Patients taking oral anticoagulants and requiring oral surgery should have the international normalized ratio (INR) measured the day of the procedure.

Fatmah Alhendi

Goals of the dental management of patients with active hepatitis B is to stabilize the patient until the active liver infection subsides and to defer all dental treatments until recovery. If treatment cannot be deferred during the active stage of the disease, consultation with the patient's physician is necessary to obtain information to avoid excessive bleeding, infection, or adverse drug reactions. Dental treatments of such patients should be carried out in an isolated operation room with adherence to the standard precautions to prevent cross-infection. An effective vaccine against hepatitis B is available; all health care workers should be fully vaccinated.

Fatmah Alhendi

Dental management of patients with alcoholic liver disease (ALD) depends on the understanding of the systemic effects of liver disease on the body's various systems. ALD can affect normal hemostatic functions by affecting platelets and coagulation factors resulting in prolonged postoperative bleeding. Given these facts, a complete blood count, liver function test, and coagulation profile should be requested before oral surgical procedures. Because the liver is an organ for drug metabolism and detoxification, liver disease may cause increased or decreased drug metabolism and hence alteration of drugs effectiveness and/or increase toxicity. Prophylactic antibiotics may be required to prevent serious infections.

Anwar A. AlMuzaini

Dentists should consult with the patient's hepatologist to obtain the most recent medical records with liver function tests and a coagulation panel. In the absence of severe liver dysfunction and with good medical management, dentists may proceed with treatment. Isolated prolongation of prothrombin time does not reflect a risk of bleeding and other coagulation parameters should be assessed. Amide local anesthesia can be safely administered and bleeding is controlled by local hemostatic measures and minimizing trauma. Other aspects of dental treatment that may require modification include the adjustment of doses of certain drugs metabolized by the liver.

Anwar A. AlMuzaini

When a patient with chronic liver disease due to a hepatitis C virus infection presents with a dental emergency, it is important to identify whether the patient is under good medical management, if severe liver dysfunction exists, or if the patient is with active hepatitis. If records are not available, contacting the patient's physician to obtain the necessary information is prudent. If the source of infection is odontogenic, extraction should not be delayed. Patients with stable chronic liver disease can safely undergo dental extractions with some modifications to the dental treatment plan.

DENTAL CLINICS OF NORTH AMERICA

THE CLINICS ARE AVAILABLE ONLINE!
Access your subscription at:
www.theclinics.com

Preface

Clinical Decisions in Medically Complex Dental Patients, Part I

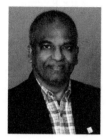 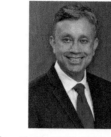

Mel Mupparapu, DMD, MDS   Andres Pinto, DMD, MPH, MBA, MSCE
Editors

When confronted with a patient who has significant comorbid medical conditions, the dental practitioner often faces the questions:

"To treat or not to treat?"; "Should I wait a bit longer?"; "Is this patient medically stable for treatment?"; "Should I refer this patient out?" Ultimately, the decision to proceed with treatment depends on the dental practitioner's comfort level, developed through prior training, knowledge, and experience. This "Clinical Decisions in Medically Complex Dental Patients, Part I" issue will come in handy when dealing with such situations. The medical scenarios are spread out in the two-part *Dental Clinics of North America* series. This first part covers several medical complexities, including diabetes, hypertension, stroke, asthma, cystic fibrosis, stem cell transplantation, human papillomavirus–related oropharyngeal cancer, and AV malformation in the jaws. In addition, the scenarios use comorbid conditions commonly noted among dental patients, such as medial arterial sclerosis, hemophilia, and von Willebrand disease. A host of situations simulating the presentation of medical complexity, including HIV infection, depression, neutropenia, emphysema, frequent mucosal pain, and red and white lesions, are included in this issue. The dental practitioner must know when to begin dental treatment in the wake of critical medical conditions, including early and severe end-stage renal disease, patients with active hepatitis B, alcoholic liver disease, end-stage liver disease, and chronic liver disease with oral infections. All of these topics are covered with individualized practical scenarios. This *Dental Clinics of North America* issue also covers medical emergencies, such as syncope, dental anxiety, history of myocardial infarction with coronary stent presenting with angina, foreign body aspiration, allergies to latex, penicillin, and local anesthetics, and other medically related conditions. The goal of these scenarios is to familiarize the dental practitioner with each medical condition so that when presented with

Dent Clin N Am 67 (2023) xix–xx
https://doi.org/10.1016/j.cden.2023.04.001
0011-8532/23/© 2023 Published by Elsevier Inc.

such a patient in real time, the condition is recognized, and treatment is safely provided, or a prompt referral is made.

We used generic names for medications so that audiences worldwide may understand them without worrying about trade names that differ from country to country, which often need clarification. Each case has keywords, key points, a synopsis, a medical scenario, a dental management decision with justification, and clinical care points. This format helps get the point across and justifies the treatment decision.

The authors and coauthors come from all across the globe, and we would like to thank them and their families with a deep appreciation for having taken the time to contribute to this *Dental Clinics of North America* issue.

We want to thank our families for their indirect contribution with their patience while we performed our obligations as editors. We enjoyed every bit of editing the articles.

Finally, we thank Elsevier, publishers of the *Dental Clinics of North America*, for their trust in our efforts to bring this issue in a format we thought would best serve dental practitioners, medical and dental residents, and dental students. We want to thank John Vassallo, the Associate Publisher of the *Dental Clinics of North America*, for his encouragement and approval of this format, and Anngie Posedio, our Developmental Editor from Reed Elsevier, Philippines, for her enthusiasm and abundant energy in putting together this issue. No issue moves forward without the production team's hard work. We thank the data administrators and the production team specialists for their help in making sure that the material is put together accurately.

We owe everything to our patients, as they are our teachers in the real world while we attempt to treat them. We would like to dedicate this issue to them.

Mel Mupparapu, DMD, MDS
University of Pennsylvania School of Dental Medicine
Philadelphia, PA 19104, USA

Andres Pinto, DMD, MPH, MBA, MSCE
School of Dental Medicine
Case Western Reserve University
Cleveland, OH 44106, USA

E-mail addresses:
mmd@upenn.edu (M. Mupparapu)
andres.pinto@case.edu (A. Pinto)

Scaling and Root Planing in a Patient with Atherosclerosis, Arrhythmia, and Anticoagulation

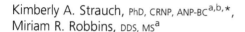

Kimberly A. Strauch, PhD, CRNP, ANP-BC[a,b,*],
Miriam R. Robbins, DDS, MS[a]

KEYWORDS

- Myocardial infarction • Coronary artery disease • Atrial fibrillation
- Direct oral anticoagulants • Dental management • Scaling and root planing

KEY POINTS

- Elective dental care should be avoided for the first 30 days following either a cardiac event (myocardial infarction) or cardiac surgery (percutaneous coronary intervention [PCI]).
- There is no indication for antibiotic prophylaxis in patients with a history of PCI.
- Both antiplatelet and direct oral anticoagulant therapy can be safely continued for low-to-medium risk dental procedures because the risk of bleeding is low.
- Any decision to alter a patient's antithrombotic regimen in order to proceed with dental care should be made in consultation with the prescribing health-care provider.
- Use of local anesthetics with vasoconstrictors among patients with a history of MI and atrial fibrillation should be limited to prevent systemic absorption and adverse cardiac effects.

MEDICAL SCENARIO

A 72-year-old man presents for scaling and root planing (SRP). His medical history is significant for a myocardial infarction (MI) 5 months ago in which he underwent successful percutaneous coronary intervention (PCI). He also has a history of atrial fibrillation (AF) that is currently controlled with medications. He is taking apixaban, clopidogrel, metoprolol succinate, lisinopril, and atorvastatin. He has a previous history of tobacco use but quit 15 years ago. He reports that lately he has noticed that his gums bleed very easily when

[a] Department of Oral Medicine, The University of Pennsylvania School of Dental Medicine, Care Center for Persons with Disabilities, 240 South 40th Street, Philadelphia, PA 19104, USA;
[b] The University of Pennsylvania School of Nursing, Claire M. Fagin Hall, 418 Curie Boulevard, Philadelphia, PA 19104, USA
* Corresponding author.
E-mail address: kstrauch@upenn.edu

Dent Clin N Am 67 (2023) 393–396
https://doi.org/10.1016/j.cden.2023.02.003
0011-8532/23/© 2023 Elsevier Inc. All rights reserved.

brushing his teeth. He admits to not always brushing twice a day and infrequently flosses. On examination, his extraoral soft tissue examination is within normal limits. Intraoral soft tissue examination is significant for generalized gingival erythema, moderate plaque and calculus accumulations, and bleeding on probing. Vital signs today are 160/84 with a pulse of 74, regular rate and rhythm. He has no known drug allergies.

DENTAL MANAGEMENT DECISION AND JUSTIFICATION

Coronary artery disease (CAD) is the most common type of heart disease in the United States and is caused by a buildup of plaque in the arteries that supply blood to the heart.[1] Overtime, this buildup can lead to arterial narrowing and partial or complete occlusion of coronary blood flow. Typical symptoms include chest pain or discomfort (angina), weakness, lightheadedness, nausea, diaphoresis, pain radiating to the arm or shoulder, and shortness of breath.[1] Risk factors for CAD include being overweight or obese, physical inactivity, poor diet, tobacco use, hypertension, diabetes, and family history of CAD (particularly in a close family member who was diagnosed with CAD at the age of 50 years or younger).[1] Conventional medical treatment of individuals who have had a MI include the initiation of an oral beta blocker, angiotensin inhibitor (angiotensin-converting enzyme inhibitor or angiotensin receptor blocker), antiplatelet agent (aspirin unless contraindicated), high-intensity statin, and nitrates as needed.[2] Some individuals with CAD have indications for combined antiplatelet and anticoagulation therapy. AF, venous thromboembolism, and valvular heart disease are the most common indications for oral anticoagulation. Individuals who require dual anticoagulant and antiplatelet therapy are a clinical challenge with regard to the need to balance the risks and benefits of intensive antithrombotic therapy. Direct oral anticoagulants (DOACs) are preferred for individuals with AF due to their superiority for stroke prevention and lower rates of major bleeding and intracranial hemorrhage compared with warfarin.[3]

Medically complex patients are frequently encountered by dental providers. Of particular concern is the risk of adverse systemic complications resulting from dental treatment, including the impact of medical conditions on dental outcomes. Current recommendations for safe and effective dental management for selected medical conditions, including CAD and AF, are suboptimal due to limited evidence, conflicting conclusions, or both.[4] Previously, it was recommended that no elective dental procedures be performed for the first 6 months following either an MI and/or PCI. More current recommendations suggest that elective care be avoided for the first 30 days following either a cardiac event or cardiac surgery.[5] Once the patient has been reevaluated by their cardiologist or cardiac surgeon and has been found to be stable, routine dental care can be provided. Additionally, there is no indication for antibiotic prophylaxis in patients with a history of PCI.

Patients with AF are at increased risk of having ischemic events during stressful dental treatment or when excessive local anesthesia with a vasoconstrictor is administered. A review of the patient's medical history, review of systems for active cardiac symptoms, and confirming that the patient has taken all of his prescribed medications should be the first step before any dental treatment. Vital signs, including blood pressure and pulse, should be obtained before all dental procedures. Short midday appointments with adequate stress management are usually preferable because the risk of an ischemic event is greatest during the first few hours of daily activity.[6] Sudden positional changes should be avoided to prevent orthostatic hypotension. Obtaining profound anesthesia is essential because pain during a dental procedure can cause endogenous catecholamine release that can cause cardiovascular stimulation. Local anesthetics with vasoconstrictors limited to 0.034 mg of epinephrine with a slow injection technique and proper aspiration can prevent systemic absorption of the vasoconstrictor and limit adverse cardiac effects.

The risks of stopping or reducing antithrombotic regimens (thromboembolism, stroke, MI) far outweigh the consequences of prolonged bleeding, which can be controlled with local measures. According to the current available evidence, both antiplatelet and DOAC therapy can be safely continued for low-to-medium risk dental procedures (simple restorations, local anesthetic administration, supragingival scaling, extractions of up to 3 teeth in the same quadrant, and minor gingival surgery) because the involved risk of bleeding is low. Most cases of perioperative or postoperative bleeding can be managed by minimizing the surgical trauma, obtaining primary closure of the wound with sutures, applying firm pressure with moistened gauze for 15 to 30 minutes, and using local hemostatic measures.[7–9] Careful postoperative instructions should be given, including to avoid rinsing or spitting for the first 24 hours, application of pressure with moistened gauze if bleeding or oozing occurs, and avoidance of nonsteroidal anti-inflammatory drugs (NSAIDs) for postoperative pain relief. Any decision to alter a patient's antithrombotic regimen should be made in consultation with the prescribing health-care provider. If necessary, the DOAC can be held the night before (if taken once a day) and the morning of the procedure (if taken twice a day) and restarted that night. Due to a significantly longer half-life, clopidogrel needs to be stopped 4 days before invasive dental procedures in order to see a clinically significant reversal.[9]

Periodontitis and poor oral health have been proposed as an etiologic or modifying risk factor in cardiovascular disease. Although the exact pathophysiology has not been fully identified, there is evidence that bacteria from the oral cavity can directly have a negative effect on existing cardiovascular damage as well as worsening systemic risk factors for cardiovascular disease. Additionally, chronic inflammation seen with periodontitis causes increased circulating levels of host inflammatory mediators (C-reactive proteins, interleukin-1β, interleukin-6, and tumor necrosis factor-α) that exacerbate cardiovascular disease directly.[10] To date, there is no evidence to prove that treatment of periodontal disease will mitigate or prevent cardiovascular disease. However, establishing and maintaining good oral health, including instituting an aggressive prevention plan to remove causative bacterial agents and treating periodontal disease may play a pivotal role in preventing future cardiovascular morbidity and mortality.[11,12]

CLINICS CARE POINTS

- Once the patient has been reevaluated by their cardiologist or cardiac surgeon and has been found to be stable, routine dental care can be provided. Consult the cardiologist or cardiac surgeon if there are concerns about anticoagulation use and planned dental care in advance of invasive procedures.

- A review of the patient's medical history, review of systems for active cardiac symptoms, and confirming that the patient has taken all of his prescribed medications should be the first step before any dental treatment.

- Vital signs, including blood pressure and pulse, should be obtained before all dental procedures. Sudden positional changes should be avoided to prevent orthostatic hypotension.

- Short midday appointments with adequate stress management are preferable because the risk of an ischemic event is greatest during the first few hours of daily activity.

- Obtaining profound anesthesia is essential because pain during a dental procedure can cause endogenous catecholamine release that can cause cardiovascular stimulation.

DISCLOSURE

Author has no conflicts of interest to disclose.

REFERENCES

1. Centers for Disease Control and Prevention. Coronary artery disease (CAD). Available at: https://www.cdc.gov/heartdisease/coronary_ad.htm. Accessed September 26, 2022.
2. Reeder GS, Kennedy HL. Overview of the nonacute management of ST-elevation myocardial infarction. In Dardas TF, ed. UpToDate; 2022. Available at: https://www.uptodate.com/contents/overview-of-the-nonacute-management-of-st-elevation-myocardial-infarction. Accessed September 26, 2022.
3. Sarafoff N, Homes DR Jr. Coronary artery disease patients requiring combined anticoagulant and antiplatelet therapy. In Parikh N, ed. UpToDate; 2022. Available at: https://www.uptodate.com/contents/coronary-artery-disease-patients-requiring-combined-anticoagulant-and-antiplatelet-therapy. Accessed September 26, 2022.
4. Napeñas JJ, Kujan O, Arduino PG, et al. World Workshop on Oral Medicine VI: Controversies regarding dental management of medically complex patients: assessment of current recommendations. Oral Surg Oral Med Oral Pathol Oral Radiol 2015;120(2):207–26.
5. Fleisher LA, Fleischmann KE, Auerbach AD, et al. 2014 ACC/AHA guideline on perioperative cardiovascular evaluation and management of patients undergoing noncardiac surgery: a report of the American College of Cardiology/American Heart Association Task Force on practice guidelines. J Am Coll Cardiol 2014; 64(22):e77–137.
6. Chaudhry S, Jaiswal R, Sachdeva S. Dental Considerations in Cardiovascular Patients: A Practical Perspective. Indian Heart J 2016;68:572–5.
7. Lusk KA, Snoga JL, Benitez RM, et al. Management of Direct-Acting Oral Anticoagulants Surrounding Dental Procedures with Low-to-Moderate Risk of Bleeding. J Pharm Pract 2018;31:202–7.
8. Kumbhani DJ, Cannon CP, Beavers CJ, et al. 2020 ACC Expert Consensus Decision Pathway for Anticoagulant and Antiplatelet Therapy in Patients with Atrial Fibrillation or Venous Thromboembolism Undergoing Percutaneous Coronary Intervention or With Atherosclerotic Cardiovascular Disease: A Report of the American College of Cardiology Solution Set Oversight Committee. J Am Coll Cardiol 2021;77(5):629–58.
9. Ockerman A, Bornstein MM, Leung YY, et al. Incidence of bleeding after minor oral surgery in patients on dual antiplatelet therapy: a systematic review and meta-analysis. Int J Oral Maxillofac Surg 2020;49(1):90–8.
10. Zardawi F, Gul S, Abdulkareem A, et al. Association Between Periodontal Disease and Atherosclerotic Cardiovascular Diseases: Revisited. Front Cardiovasc Med 2021;7:579–625.
11. Larvin H, Kang J, Aggarwal VR, et al. Risk of incident cardiovascular disease in people with periodontal disease: A systematic review and meta-analysis. Clin Exp Dent Res 2021;7(1):109–22.
12. Rahimi A, Afshari Z. Periodontitis and cardiovascular disease: A literature review. ARYA Atheroscler 2021;17(5):1–8.

Restorative Treatment in a Patient with Symptomatic Valvular and Structural Heart Disease

Kimberly A. Strauch, PhD, CRNP, ANP-BC[a,b,*],
Miriam R. Robbins, DDS, MS[a]

KEYWORDS

- Left ventricular hypertrophy • Reduced ejection fraction • Dyspnea
- Aortic valve replacement • Dental management • Restorative treatment

KEY POINTS

- Individuals with acutely decompensated heart failure (HF) require prompt intervention, and any elective dental care should be postponed until symptoms are stable.
- Vasoactive agents should be used cautiously in individuals with advanced HF.
- Individuals on anticoagulation for valvular replacement should not be discontinued and most dental procedures can be safely performed with an international normalized ratio up to 3.5.
- Patients with a history of valve replacement surgery should receive infective endocarditis prophylaxis for all dental procedures.

MEDICAL SCENARIO

A 79-year-old woman presents for restorative treatment. Her medical history is significant for a history of aortic stenosis with concomitant left ventricular (LV) hypertrophy and New York Heart Association (NYHA)[1,2] Functional Class II, Stage B HF with reduced ejection fraction (HFrEF). Her aortic valve was replaced with a mechanical valve one year ago. Her current ejection fraction is 37%. She is taking warfarin daily, nebivolol, furosemide, valsartan, and atorvastatin. She reports a history of hives with penicillin. As she sits down in the dental chair, you notice that both of her ankles are slightly swollen. She asks you not to lay the chair back too far because she has trouble breathing when she is fully supine. Her blood pressure today is 130/68 with a pulse of 74, regular rate and rhythm.

Neither author has any conflicts of interest to disclose.
[a] Department of Oral Medicine, The University of Pennsylvania School of Dental Medicine, Care Center for Persons with Disabilities, 240 South 40th Street, Philadelphia, PA 19104, USA;
[b] The University of Pennsylvania School of Nursing, Claire M. Fagin Hall, 418 Curie Boulevard, Philadelphia, PA 19104, USA
* Corresponding author.
E-mail address: kstrauch@upenn.edu

https://doi.org/10.1016/j.cden.2023.02.004
0011-8532/23/© 2023 Elsevier Inc. All rights reserved.
dental.theclinics.com

DENTAL MANAGEMENT DECISION AND JUSTIFICATION

HF is a complex clinical syndrome characterized by the objective and subjective presence of current or previous symptoms, such as dyspnea and fatigue, and evidence of cardiac dysfunction as the underlying cause of these symptoms.[1–3] From a hemodynamic perspective, HF creates a scenario whereby the heart cannot pump enough blood to keep up with the body's demands or can only do so at the expense of higher than normal filling pressures.[3] Consequently, HF is the result of structural or functional cardiac disorders that impair the ability of the ventricle(s) to fill with and eject blood. Common causes of HF include hypertension, history of myocardial infarction or obstructive lesions of the great vessels, valvular heart disease, pericardial disease, and right or LV dysfunction.[3] There is no gold standard to diagnose HF. Rather, diagnosis is made based on a thorough history, physical examination, laboratory data, and imaging studies.

HF caused by LV dysfunction is commonly categorized according to LV ejection fraction (LVEF), which is measured via echocardiogram. The echocardiogram is a noninvasive imaging study that provides clinicians with details about the structure and function of the heart. LVEF refers to the amount of blood pumped out of the ventricles with each contraction. The ejection fraction in a normally functioning heart is 50% to 70%.[3] HF with LVEF of 40% or lesser is known as HFrEF.[3] HF with LVEF of 41% to 49% is HF with midrange ejection fraction.[3] HF with LVEF of 50% or greater may be caused by HF with preserved ejection fraction or a cardiomyopathy (restrictive, hypertrophic, or noncompaction).[3]

Identification of HF symptoms by the dental provider will be key to providing safe and effective care. Acute and subacute presentations of HF (days to weeks of onset) are characterized by shortness of breath at rest and/or with exertion, orthopnea, paroxysmal nocturnal dyspnea, and palpitations with or without lightheadedness.[3] Acutely decompensated individuals require prompt intervention and any elective dental care should be postponed until symptoms are stable. The presentation of chronic HF (ongoing for months) is one of compensation due to the slow, insidious onset of symptoms. Fatigue, anorexia, peripheral edema, and abdominal distention may be more pronounced than dyspnea, which may be more exertional and subtle in nature.[3]

Dental management of patients with compensated HF includes shorter appointments to reduce stress. For patients with NYHA Class I or II HF, up to 0.034 mg of local anesthetic with 1:100,000 epinephrine can be safely used.[4] Vasoconstrictors should be used cautiously in NYHA Class III or IV patients and in patients taking digoxin. Patients should be treated with the head elevated in an upright position at least 30° to 90° in the dental chair to decrease the chance of pulmonary edema. Supplemental oxygen may be used for patients with notable dyspnea. Vital signs should be closely monitored and appointments terminated if the patient becomes fatigued, severely short of breath, or hypoxic.

Individuals with mechanical valve repairs require lifelong anticoagulation with a vitamin K antagonist (VKA; such as warfarin) to reduce the risk of thromboembolism. Warfarin requires targeted dosing and monitoring using the international normalized ratio (INR). The standard INR target for individuals with mechanical aortic valves is 3.0 ± 0.5 units.[5] Frequency of monitoring depends on therapeutic levels. At minimum, the INR should be checked monthly. It will be important to have the most recent INR on file before elective or emergent dental care to minimize bleeding risks that may occur with treatment. Current evidence shows that most dental procedures, including moderately invasive surgery (tooth extractions, biopsy, periodontal treatment) can be safely done with an INR up to 3.5, using local hemostatic measures.[6,7] Discontinuation of anticoagulant therapy puts the patient at significantly higher risk of a thromboembolic event[8] and exceeds the risk of significant bleeding complications if anticoagulation is continued.

Patients with a history of valve replacement surgery should receive infective endocarditis prophylaxis for all dental procedures that involve manipulation of gingival or periapical tissue or perforation of the oral mucosa (**Table 1**). This includes all prosthetic cardiac valves (including transcatheter-implanted prostheses and homografts) as well as cardiac valve repair with prosthetic materials, such as annuloplasty rings and chords.[9] Because it may cause more frequent or severe side effects (ie, *Clostridium difficile* infection), clindamycin is no longer recommended for antibiotic prophylaxis for dental procedures unless there are no other viable options.[9] The patient in this case came prepared by taking oral antibiotic prophylaxis one hour before her appointment as prescribed by her cardiologist. Additionally, people with underlying cardiac conditions that put them at increased risk of developing infectious endocarditis should be strongly encouraged to establish and maintain optimal oral health through daily oral hygiene coupled with routine dental visits to decrease the chance of bacterial seeding from the oral cavity to the heart.[10]

Table 1
Adult and pediatric prophylactic antibiotic regimens for the prevention of dental-related infective endocarditis

	Adult Oral Medications & Doses	Adult Parenteral Medications, Routes, and Doses	Pediatric Oral Medications & Doses	Pediatric Parenteral Medications, Routes, and Doses
No Penicillin Allergy	Amoxicillin 2 g	Ampicillin 2 g IM or IV OR Cefazolin or Ceftriaxone 1 g IM or IV	Amoxicillin 50 mg/kg	Ampicillin 50 mg/kg IM or IV OR Cefazolin or Ceftriaxone 50 mg/kg IM or IV
Known Penicillin Allergy	[a,b]Cephalexin 2 g OR Doxycycline 100 mg OR Azithromycin or Clarithromycin 500 mg	Cefazolin or Ceftriaxone 1 g IM or IV	[a,b]Cephalexin 50 mg/kg OR Doxycycline <45 kg = 2.2 mg/kg ≥45 kg = 100 mg OR Azithromycin or Clarithromycin 15 mg/kg	Cefazolin or [b]Ceftriaxone 50 mg/kg IM or IV

Abbreviations: IM, intramuscular; IV, intravenous.

All doses are a single dose administered 30-60 minutes prior to dental treatment.

Clindamycin is no longer recommended for antibiotic prophylaxis unless there are no other options.

[a] Other first- or second-generation oral cephalosporins in equivalent adult or pediatric dosages acceptable

[b] Cephalosporins should not be prescribed in an individual with a history of anaphylaxis, angioedema, or urticaria with penicillin or ampicillin.

Data from Wilson WR, Gewitz M, Lockhart PB, et al. Prevention of Viridans Group Streptococcal Infective Endocarditis: A Scientific Statement from the American Heart Association. Circulation. 2021;143(20):e963–e978.

CLINICS CARE POINTS

- Supplemental oxygen may be used for patients with notable dyspnea. Vital signs should be closely monitored and appointments terminated if the patient becomes fatigued, severely short of breath, or hypoxic.
- Patients with compensated HF require shorter appointments to reduce stress.
- Patients should be treated with their head elevated in an upright position at least 30-90 degrees in the dental chair to decrease the chance of pulmonary edema and shortness of breath.
- Verify that the patient has come prepared to the appointment by taking prescribed oral antibiotic prophylaxis one hour before the appointment.
- Verify any prescribed anticoagulation regimens, consider risks vs. benefits of planned dental care, and if indicated, obtain copies of most recent labs (i.e. PT/INR) prior to the appointment.

REFERENCES

1. Dolgin M, Fox AC, Gorlin R, et al. New York Heart Association. Criteria Committee. Nomenclature and criteria for diagnosis of diseases of the heart and great vessels. 9th edition. Boston, MA: Lippincott Williams and Wilkins; 1994.
2. American Heart Association. Classes of heart failure. Available at: https://www.heart.org/en/health-topics/heart-failure/what-is-heart-failure/classes-of-heart-failure. Accessed September 23, 2022.
3. Colucci WS, Borlaug BA. Heart failure: clinical manifestations and diagnosis in adults. In: Dardas TF, editor. UpToDate. 2022. Available at: https://www.uptodate.com/contents/heart-failure-clinical-manifestations-and-diagnosis-in-adults. Accessed September 23, 2022.
4. Elad S, Admon D, Kedmi M, et al. The cardiovascular effect of local anesthesia with articaine plus 1:200,000 adrenalin versus lidocaine plus 1:100,000 adrenalin in medically compromised cardiac patients: a prospective, randomized, double blinded study. Oral Surg Oral Med Oral Pathol Oral Radiol Endod 2008;105(6): 725–30.
5. Otto CM, Nishimura RA, Bonow RO, et al. ACC/AHA guideline for the management of patients with valvular heart disease: a report of the american college of cardiology/american heart association joint committee on clinical practice guidelines. Circulation 2021;143:e72.
6. Hong CH, Napenas JJ, Brennan MT, et al. Risk of postoperative bleeding after dental procedures in patients on warfarin: A Retrospective Study. Oral Surg Oral Med Oral Pathol Oral Radio 2012;114:464–8.
7. AAOM clinical practice statement: subject: management of patients on warfarin therapy. Oral Surg Oral Med Oral Pathol Oral Radiol 2016;122(6):702–4.
8. Wahl MJ, Pinto A, Kilham J, et al. Dental surgery in anticoagulated patients–stop the interruption. Oral Surg Oral Med Oral Pathol Oral Radiol 2015;119(2): 136–57.
9. Wilson WR, Gewitz M, Lockhart PB, et al. Prevention of viridans group streptococcal infective endocarditis: a scientific statement from the American Heart Association. Circulation 2021;143(20):e963–78.

10. Wilson W, Taubert KA, Gewitz M, et al. Prevention of infective endocarditis: guidelines from the American Heart Association: a guideline from the American Heart Association rheumatic fever, endocarditis and kawasaki disease committee, council on cardiovascular disease in the young, and the council on clinical cardiology, council on cardiovascular surgery and anesthesia, and the quality of care and outcomes research interdisciplinary working group. J Am Dent Assoc 2008; 139(Suppl):3S–24S.

Crown Preparation in a Patient with Hypertension and Type 2 Diabetes Mellitus

Miriam R. Robbins, DDS, MS[a],*, Kimberly A. Strauch, PhD, ANP-BC[a,b]

KEYWORDS

- Hypertension • High blood pressure • Hyperglycemia • Diabetes
- Crown preparation • Dental management

KEY POINTS

- There is no evidence to support having an arbitrary point-of-care glucose cutoff point of 200 mg/dL for dental care.
- Individuals with poor glycemic control can be prone to delayed wound healing secondary to the microvascular changes and impaired host defense mechanisms.
- Glycemic control has not been shown to affect the rate of post-extraction epithelialization and subsequent healing.
- Gingivitis, periodontitis, and associated bone loss independent of plaque accumulation are associated with poorly controlled diabetes.
- Gingival hyperplasia is a common and often overlooked side effect of people taking calcium channel blockers for the treatment of hypertension.

MEDICAL SCENARIO

A 57-year-old man presents to the dental office for crown preparation and impression on a lower right molar. He has no acute dental complaints. His medical history is significant for hypertension, hyperlipidemia, and diabetes mellitus type 2 (DM2). His medications include nifedipine, losartan, glipizide, dulaglutide, atorvastatin, and aspirin. He has no known drug allergies. On examination, his vital signs are 160/94 (left arm, sitting) and 158/92 (right arm, sitting) with a pulse of 80 beats per minute with a regular rate and rhythm. His point-of-care (POC) glucose is 197. On questioning, he states that he had a large coffee with two sugars and a donut about 1 hour before his appointment. A review of his recent blood work shows a hemoglobin A1C of 8% and a creatinine of 1.1. His

[a] Department of Oral Health, Care Center for Persons with Disabilities, The University of Pennsylvania School of Dental Medicine, 240 South 40th Street, Philadelphia, PA 19104, USA;
[b] The University of Pennsylvania School of Nursing, Claire M. Fagin Hall, 418 Curie Boulevard, Philadelphia, PA 19104, USA
* Corresponding author.
E-mail address: mrrobb@upenn.edu

Dent Clin N Am 67 (2023) 403–406
https://doi.org/10.1016/j.cden.2023.02.005
0011-8532/23/© 2023 Elsevier Inc. All rights reserved.

dental.theclinics.com

diabetes and hypertension are currently managed by his primary care provider. The extraoral soft tissue examination is within normal limits. The intraoral soft tissue examination reveals generalized gingival erythema with periodontal pockets ranging from 3 to 6 mm with bleeding on probing.

DENTAL MANAGEMENT DECISION AND JUSTIFICATION

The dental team is an important part of improving a patient's metabolic control by achieving and maintaining optimal oral health, thus reducing the morbidity associated with diabetes. Management of the diabetic dental patient should focus on the delivery of comprehensive dental care with an emphasis on maintaining periodontal health. Obtaining a through medical history and review of systems, including information pertaining to the degree of glycemic control, history of hypoglycemic episodes, and identification of comorbidities is essential before beginning dental treatment. Care should be taken to deliver dental treatment with minimal disruption of metabolic homeostasis.

DM2 is a metabolic disorder characterized by hyperglycemia often due to inappropriate insulin secretion and/or action. Diagnosis of DM2 is based on the following criteria: (1) a fasting plasma glucose greater than 126 mg/dL; (2) a hemoglobin A1C $\geq$ 6.5%; (3) a random plasma glucose $\geq$200 mg/dL 2 hours after eating; or (4) a random plasma glucose $\geq$200 mg/dL taken at any time along with overt diabetic symptoms (polyuria, polyphagia, and polydipsia).[1] The hemoglobin A1c is an indirect measure that reflects a person's average blood glucose over approximately 3 months[2] (**Table 1**). It is the primary tool for diagnosing and assessing glycemic control. The POC or self-monitoring blood glucose value is simply a snapshot of the blood glucose at a single point in time and is influenced by a variety of factors (ie, timing of food intake, timing of medications, stressors, and acute illness). The A1C does not provide a measure of glycemic variability or hypoglycemia, which is why it is important to have a recent A1C on file so as to compare that to the POC glucose taken during the dental visit.[2] There is no evidence to support having an arbitrary POC glucose cutoff point of 200 mg/dL for dental care. Although patients with poor glycemic control can be prone

Table 1 Hemoglobin A1C and estimated average blood glucose		
A1C (%)	mg/dL	mmol/L
5	97	5.4
6	126	7.0
7	154	8.6
8	183	10.2
9	212	11.8
10	240	13.4
11	269	14.9
12	298	16.5
13	326	18.1
14	355	19.7

Note. This table lists the percentage of glycosylated hemoglobin, or Hemoglobin A1C, and the average blood sugar associated with that percentage.

Adapted from the American Diabetes Association. Standards of Medical Care in Diabetes. *Diabetes Care.* 2021;44(Suppl. 1):S73-S84; and Selvin E. Measurements of glycemic control in diabetes mellitus. In Rubinow K, ed. *UpToDate;* 2022. https://www.uptodate.com/contents/measurements-of-glycemic-control-in-diabetes-mellitus.

to delayed wound healing secondary to the microvascular changes and impaired host defense mechanisms seen, glycemic control has not been shown to affect the rate of post-extraction epithelialization and subsequent healing.[3,4] Each case must be reviewed on an individual basis to determine if dental care can proceed if the patient is not normoglycemic. An A1C of less than 7% is an acceptable target for most nonpregnant adults without a significant history of hypoglycemia.[2] Less stringent A1C targets (such as < 8%) may be appropriate for patients with limited life expectancy (such as older adults), history of severe hypoglycemia, advanced microvascular or macrovascular complications, extensive comorbid conditions, or long-standing DM2 in which the target A1C is difficult to achieve despite appropriate care/education.[2]

Periodontal diseases are chronic inflammatory processes that occur due to the prolonged presence of subgingival bacterial biofilm (dental plaque).[5] Although the etiology of periodontal diseases is multifactorial, there is a strong association between DM2 and periodontal disease,[5] often called the "sixth complication of diabetes mellitus."[6] Gingivitis, periodontitis, and associated bone loss independent of plaque accumulation are associated with poorly controlled diabetes. Dysregulation of immune function, more pathogenic bacterial flora, and microvascular disease are all thought to contribute to diabetic periodontal disease. Periodontal status should be monitored carefully in patients with diabetes and underlying disease managed aggressively. Consideration should be made to increasing recall and maintenance frequency.

Nearly half of all American adults (47% or 116 million) have a diagnosis of hypertension, which is one of the leading preventable causes of chronic disease and death.[7,8] Hypertension is defined as a systolic blood pressure greater than 130 mm Hg and a diastolic blood pressure greater than 80 mm Hg and is based on the average of two or more readings taken at two separate visits.[6] The dental team plays an important role in the identification of hypertension and referral to appropriate follow-up care in instances when the blood pressure is high. Stimulants (ie, caffeine, prescription and nonprescription stimulants), nicotine, stress or emotions, "white coat syndrome," fear or anxiety, pain, weight gain, and forgetting to take prescribed medications are some of the key reasons individuals may have high blood pressure. Because this individual is taking nifedipine—a calcium channel blocker—it will be important to assess for gingival hyperplasia, a common and often overlooked side effect of this medication class.[9] If gingival hyperplasia is observed and all other causes ruled out, it may be prudent to contact the prescribing provider to discuss switching the calcium channel blocker to another antihypertensive medication.

CLINICS CARE POINTS

- Patients with diabetes are more prone to oral infections, especially periodontal disease. Regular dental checkups and good oral hygiene practices are important to prevent complications.

- Oral health care providers should be aware of the patient's blood glucose levels before and during dental procedures, as poorly controlled blood sugar levels can increase the risk of infections and delay wound healing.

- It is important to take and record the patient's blood pressure before and after the procedure.

- The use of epinephrine-containing local anesthesia is generally safe in patients with controlled hypertension, but caution should be taken in those with severe hypertension or who are taking certain medications.

- Good communication between the dentist and the patient's healthcare team is essential for managing the patient's blood sugar levels and blood pressures during dental procedures.
- Dentists should be aware of the patient's hypertension medications, as some can cause xerostomia (dry mouth) or gingival overgrowth, which can affect oral health.

DISCLOSURE

Neither author has any conflicts of interest to disclose.

REFERENCES

1. American Diabetes Association. Understanding A1C: Diagnosis. Available at: https://diabetes.org/diabetes/a1c/diagnosis. Accessed September 18, 2022.
2. American Diabetes Association. Standards of Medical Care in Diabetes. Diabetes Care 2021;44(Suppl. 1):S73–84.
3. Aronovich S, Skope LW, Kelly JP, et al. The relationship of glycemic control to the outcomes of dental extractions. J Oral Maxillofac Surg 2010;68(12):2955–61.
4. Joshipura K. Glycemic control is not related to postextraction healing in patients with diabetes. J Evid Based Dent Pract 2011;11(4):187–8.
5. Bascones-Martinez A, Gonzalez-Febles J, Sanz-Esporrin J. Diabetes and periodontal disease. Review of the literature. Am J Dent 2014;27(2):63–7.
6. Lamster IB, Lalla E, Borgnakke WS, et al. The relationship between oral health and diabetes mellitus. J Am Dent Assoc 2008;139(Suppl):S19–24.
7. Centers for Disease Control and Prevention (CDC). Hypertension cascade: hypertension prevalence, treatment and control estimates among US adults aged 18 Years and older applying the criteria from the American college of cardiology and American heart association's 2017 hypertension guideline—NHANES 2015–2018. Atlanta (GA): US Department of Health and Human Services; 2021. Available at: https://www.cdc.gov/bloodpressure/facts.htm. Accessed September 18, 2022.
8. James PA, Oparil S, Carter BL, et al. 2014 Evidence-Based Guideline for the Management of High Blood Pressure in Adults: Report from the Panel Members Appointed to the Eighth Joint National Committee (JNC 8). JAMA 2014;311(5):507–20.
9. Fardal O, Lygre H. Management of periodontal disease in patients using calcium channel blockers - gingival overgrowth, prescribed medications, treatment responses and added treatment costs. J Clin Periodontol 2015;42(7):640–6.

Treatment of a Mandibular Abscess in a Patient with Coronary Artery Disease and Intermittent Angina

Miriam R. Robbins, DDS, MS[a],*, Kimberly A. Strauch, PhD, ANP-BC[a,b]

KEYWORDS

- Coronary artery disease • Coronary artery bypass graft • Angina • Obesity
- Mandibular abscess

KEY POINTS

- The dental environment can increase the likelihood of an anginal attack due to fear, pain, or anxiety associated with dental care.
- Patients at risk for or with known anginal symptoms should be encouraged to bring their usual anti-anginal therapy with them to all dental appointments.
- Coronary artery bypass graft surgery is not associated with a long-term risk of infection and therefore, antibiotic prophylaxis among this population is not necessary.
- Although rare, interactions between epinephrine and nonselective beta-blockers can lead to significant hypertension and reflex bradycardia, and local anesthetics with epinephrine should be limited.
- Antiplatelet and anticoagulant medications should be continued, and local hemostatic measures should be used to control bleeding.

INTRODUCTION

A patient with a history of coronary artery bypass graft surgery four months ago with a history of intermittent angina and morbid obesity presents with a mandibular abscess.

MEDICAL SCENARIO

A 63-year-old man presents for an emergency appointment with a 24-hour history of left mandibular swelling and 10/10 pain. He reports that he has had tooth pain in the

[a] Department of Oral Health, The University of Pennsylvania School of Dental Medicine, Care Center for Persons with Disabilities, 240 South 40th Street, Room 209A, Philadelphia, PA 19104, USA; [b] The University of Pennsylvania School of Nursing, Claire M. Fagin Hall, 418 Curie Boulevard, Philadelphia, PA 19104, USA
* Corresponding author.
E-mail address: mrrobb@upenn.edu

Dent Clin N Am 67 (2023) 407–410
https://doi.org/10.1016/j.cden.2023.02.006
0011-8532/23/© 2023 Elsevier Inc. All rights reserved.

dental.theclinics.com

area off and on for the past 2 weeks but the pain intensity has significantly increased since yesterday. He was unable to sleep, and the pain was unrelieved with additional strength acetaminophen. He denies any fever or chills. His medical history is significant for a 3-vessel coronary artery bypass graft (CABG) approximately 4 months ago. He also reports intermittent, substernal chest pain with exertion that is relieved by rest. He is 5'11" and weighs 270 lbs (body mass index [BMI] of 37). His medications include transdermal nitroglycerin, carvedilol, lisinopril, clopidogrel, aspirin, and atorvastatin. On examination, tooth #18 is grossly carious. There is fluctuance in the buccal vestibule and an associated fullness along the inferior border of the mandible. His blood pressure today is 134/84, pulse 66 with a regular rate and rhythm, and temperature of 98.9°F. He reports no difficulty in swallowing and examination of the floor of the mouth and oropharynx are within normal limits.

DENTAL MANAGEMENT DECISION AND JUSTIFICATION

CAD is the leading cause of death worldwide.[1] As such, the prevalence of cardiac disorders among the general population, specifically ischemic heart disease, means that dental providers will frequently encounter patients with these conditions. In fact, CAD is the most frequently cited medical condition that warrants a referral from general dental practitioners to either an outpatient cardiologist or hospital-based departments of oral and maxillo-facial surgery.[2] This reflects a pervasive concern over potential complications among cardiac patients during dental treatment.

Because cardiac disorders are common, an evaluation of the medical history is an essential first step in determining the treatment plan. It is prudent to update the medical history at every visit, which includes any changes to medications, verification of drug allergies, recent surgeries, changes in the social history, and confirmation of key nondental providers on the patient's care team. Next, a focused review of systems should be performed at every visit. In this case, it is important to assess for any signs or symptoms of stable or unstable angina. Typically, anginal pain is precipitated by factors that increase myocardial oxygen demand, which often includes physical activity or exertion, and usually resolves with rest. The dental environment can increase the likelihood of an anginal attack due to fear, pain, or anxiety associated with dental care.[3] Patients at risk for or with known anginal symptoms should be encouraged to bring their usual antianginal therapy with them to all dental appointments.[3] Oral or inhaled nitrates are the standard emergency treatment of angina. If a patient experiences anginal symptoms while in the chair, stop treatment and allow the patient to relieve the attack themselves in their usual manner (assuming they have their antianginal agent with them). Supplemental oxygen may be administered if available but this is not usually required. Common side effects of nitrates include hypotension, headache, and dizziness. They should be used as directed and vital signs should be monitored closely. After the anginal attack has passed, it will normally be safe to continue dental treatment if the patient wishes. If the chest pain is prolonged or unrelieved with antianginal agents, then the patient may be having a myocardial infarction. This is a medical emergency, and hence, emergency medical services should be called. Should the patient undergo a cardiac arrest and use of the automated external defibrillator (AED) is needed, it will be important to make sure this patient's transdermal nitroglycerin patch is not in a location where the AED pads will be attached to the body.

Because the patient recently underwent open-heart surgery, consultation with the cardiologist is advisable to ascertain cardiac stability. There is no need for antibiotic prophylaxis in this case because CABG surgery is not associated with a long-term risk of infection.[4] Vital signs should be monitored during the procedure and oxygen and nitroglycerin should be easily accessible. Care should be taken when administering a local anesthetic to the patient secondary to carvedilol (a nonselective nonselective beta-adrenergic blocking agent). Although rare, there can be a potentially significant interaction between epinephrine and nonselective beta-blockers leading to significant hypertension with a concomitant reflex bradycardia. Local anesthetics with epinephrine should be limited to not more than 0.034 mg of local anesthetic with 1:100,000 epinephrine delivered with careful aspiration to ensure that there is no intravascular delivery.[5]

The patient should be treated in a semi-Fowler's position (with the head elevated in an upright position at least 30°–60° in the dental chair) secondary to the increased BMI. There is no need to delay treatment because of the antithrombotic therapy. Recent systematic reviews found no clinically significant increased risk of postoperative bleeding complications from invasive dental procedures in patients on antiplatelet therapy.[6,7] Current literature supports the continuation of both antiplatelet and anticoagulant medications and the use of local hemostatic measures to control bleeding. The patient should be placed on an appropriate course of postoperative antibiotics and monitored carefully for resolution of his infection.

CLINICS CARE POINTS

- The key to treating patients with CAD is to understand their medical history, coordinate with their physician, and take steps to minimize risk and ensure patient comfort during dental procedures.

- Incorporating stress reduction techniques such as deep breathing exercises, music, or relaxation techniques may help reduce anxiety and improve patient comfort.

- There is no evidence to support use of antibiotic prophylaxis in patients with a history of cardiac stenting or coronary-artery bypass surgery. undergoing dental procedures.

- Judicious use of local anesthesia with epinepherine to ensure profound anesthesia is warrented but should be limited, especially for patients taking non-selective beta-blockers4. A careful review of systems, including any recent anginal events, should be done at every visit.

DISCLOSURE

Neither author has any conflicts of interest to disclose.

REFERENCES

1. World Health Organization. The top 10 causes of death. Available at: https://www.who.int/news-room/fact-sheets/detail/the-top-10-causes-of-death. Accessed September 22, 2022.
2. Absi EG, Satterthwaite J, Shepherd JP, et al. The appropriateness of referral of medically compromised dental patients to hospital. Br J Oral Maxillofac Surg 1997;35(2):133–6.
3. Jowett N, Cabot L. Patients with cardiac disease: considerations for the dental practitioner. Br Dent J 2000;189(6):297–302.
4. Wilson WR, Gewitz M, Lockhart PB, et al. Prevention of Viridans Group Streptococcal Infective Endocarditis: A Scientific Statement From the American Heart Association. Circulation 2021;143(20):e963–78 [published correction appears in

Circulation. 2021;144(9):e192] [published correction appears in Circulation. 2022 Apr 26;145(17):e868].

5. Hersh EV, Giannakopoulos H. Beta-adrenergic blocking agents and dental vaso-constrictors. Dent Clin North Am 2010;54(4):687–96.

6. Napenas JJ, Oost FC, DeGroot A, et al. Review of postoperative bleeding risk in dental patients on antiplatelet therapy. Oral Surg Oral Med Oral Pathol Oral Radiol 2013;115(4):491–9.

7. Jeske AH, Suchko GD. Lack of a scientific basis for routine discontinuation of oral anticoagulation therapy before dental treatment. J Am Dent Assoc 2003;134(11): 1492–7.

A Patient with Permanent Cardiac Pacemaker, History of Stroke Presents for an Extraction of Mandibular Molar Tooth

Miriam R. Robbins, DDS, MS[a],*, Kimberly A. Strauch, PhD, ANP-BC[a,b]

KEYWORDS

- Stroke • Cerebral vascular accident • Permanent cardiac pacemaker • Extraction
- Dental management

KEY POINTS

- Stroke survivors typically have higher rates of xerostomia and aspiration pneumonia, and overall, poorer oral health and nutritional status compared with the general population.
- Modifications to dental treatment of stroke survivors should be based on the degree of neurologic sequelae and overall medical stability.
- Patients with a permanent cardiac pacemaker (PPM) do not require antibiotic prophylaxis before dental treatment.
- It is prudent to know the brand and/or model of every patient's PPM so as not to cause unnecessary telemetry or electromagnetic interference when using ultrasonic dental equipment.

MEDICAL SCENARIO

A 61-year-old man presents for periodic examination and cleaning. His medical history is significant for a history of a right-sided cerebrovascular accident (CVA) secondary to a history of atrial fibrillation. He subsequently underwent placement of a permanent cardiac pacemaker (PPM). The CVA left him with some weakness in his left arm and hand. There were no speech or swallowing deficits. His medications include rivaroxaban, atorvastatin, metoprolol, and enalapril. The vital signs today are 130/80, pulse

Neither author has any conflicts of interest to disclose.
[a] Department of Oral Medicine, The University of Pennsylvania School of Dental Medicine, Care Center for Persons with Disabilities, 240 South 40th Street, Philadelphia, PA 19104, USA;
[b] The University of Pennsylvania School of Nursing, Claire M. Fagin Hall, 418 Curie Boulevard, Philadelphia, PA 19104, USA
* Corresponding author.
E-mail address: mrrobb@upenn.edu

Dent Clin N Am 67 (2023) 411–413
https://doi.org/10.1016/j.cden.2023.02.007
0011-8532/23/© 2023 Elsevier Inc. All rights reserved.

of 70 with an irregularly irregular rate and rhythm. He has no known drug allergies. Extraoral soft tissue exam is within normal limits. Intraoral soft tissue exam reveals moderate plaque and soft debris is present, especially on the right side with generalized bleeding on probing. There is moderate calculus buildup on the linguals of the lower anterior teeth as well as interproximally on the upper molars.

DENTAL MANAGEMENT DECISION AND JUSTIFICATION

Strokes or CVAs are the leading cause of death in the United States.[1] Strokes can be ischemic (ie, reduced or complete loss of blood flow to cerebral vessels due to atherosclerotic plaques or blood clots) or hemorrhagic (ie, ruptured cerebral vessels causing bleeding around the brain). Transient ischemic attack, or TIA, is sometimes referred to as a "mini stroke." A TIA is different from a stroke because it is a temporary and self-limited blockage of blood flow to the brain (ie, less than 5 minutes); however, it is a warning sign of impending stroke.[1] Common symptoms of stroke include unilateral facial weakness or facial drooping, trouble with speech, sudden confusion, severe headache (worst headache of life), acute changes in vision (one or both eyes), unilateral numbness or weakness in a limb or the face, and difficulty walking. Stroke symptoms are a medical emergency and require prompt intervention to prevent permanent disability or death.

Poor oral health and/or dental disease are highly prevalent among stroke survivors. Current research points to an inflammatory pathway linking poor oral health to stroke risk.[2] Stroke survivors typically have fewer teeth than individuals without stroke and often wear dentures.[3] Xerostomia is a common side effect of stroke-related medications, which can increase the risk of tooth decay, periodontal disease, and oral infections, and negatively impact denture use. Likewise, poor oral health among stroke survivors has been linked to higher rates of aspiration pneumonia,[4] reduced quality of life, and poorer nutritional status.[5] Tooth decay and periodontal disease among stroke survivors can be prevented or effectively managed with appropriate oral health behaviors; however, oral hygiene routines may be disrupted by the stroke itself and subsequent acquired physical or cognitive deficits may make regular oral hygiene more difficult.[6] Unilateral paralysis of the muscles of the face and oral cavity coupled with tongue flaccidity can lead to dysphagia and accumulation of food debris on the affected side. Muscle weakness and loss of dexterity can decrease the patient's ability to provide effective oral hygiene, especially if the person has residual physical limitations on the dominant side. It is important for the dental care team to address individual barriers related to home oral hygiene self-care and access to dental services for stroke survivors.[6]

Before initiation of treatment, the patient should be evaluated in terms of the ability to communicate and provide informed consent for treatment. If the patient's mental capacity has been affected, then determination of who has the power of attorney to consent to treatment is needed before proceeding. In general, elective dental treatment should be delayed until the patient is deemed stable from a neurologic standpoint. Modifications to treatment should be based on the degree of neurologic sequelae, including scheduling needs (ie, late morning or early afternoon appointments may be best). Vital signs should be carefully monitored. Local anesthetics with vasoconstrictors should be used carefully and limited to 0.036 mg of epinephrine. Patients with dysphagia may have reduced gag reflexes and should be seated in a semi-Fowler's or high Fowler's position (with the head elevated in an upright position at least 30–90° in the dental chair) with ongoing suction to prevent aspiration of saliva and foreign matter. Patients may need support pillows while in the chair to remain in an upright position. Chair position should be changed slowly to reduce the risk of orthostatic hypotension caused by rapid chair repositioning.[7]

PPMs are an effective treatment of a variety of bradyarrhythmias and conduction abnormalities. Cardiac pacing provides an appropriate heart rate and cardiac response to re-establish effective circulation and normalize hemodynamics otherwise compromised by a slow heart rate or conduction abnormality. Patients with a PPM do not require antibiotic prophylaxis before dental treatment but dental providers should inquire about the PPM brand and/or model. Most patients carry a wallet card to make this information readily available to their care team. Modern PPMs are bipolar and shielded which lower the risk of malfunction due to electromagnetic interference. Piezoelectric and magnetostrictive ultrasonic dental scalers, electronic pulp testers, apex locators, and curing lights cause minor telemetry interference and no adverse events in function, and thus, can be used safely in patients with shielded PPMs.[8] Monopolar electrosurgery units, however, result in clinically significant electromagnetic interference and should be avoided.

CLINICS CARE POINTS

- A thorough medical history should be obtained from the patient, including the type of pacemaker, date of implantation, and any relevant medical conditions or medications.
- Vital signs should be closely monitored prior to initiation of treatment.
- Monopolar electrosurgery units can cause electromagnetic interference and should be avoided in patients with pacemakers.
- For patients with neurologic impairment post CVA, barriers to home oral hygiene self-care should be identified and addressed to ensure the maintainence of good oral health.

REFERENCES

1. Centers for Disease Control and Prevention. Stroke. Available at: https://www.cdc.gov/stroke/index.htm. Accessed September 26, 2022.
2. Lee Y-L, Hu H-Y, Huang N, et al. Dental pro-phylaxis and periodontal treatment are protective factors to ischemic stroke. Stroke 2013;44(4):1026–30.
3. Dai r, Lam OLT, Lo ECM, et al. A systematic review and meta-analysis of clinical, microbiological, and behavioural aspects of oral health among patients with stroke. J Dent 2015;43(2):171–80.
4. Sellars C, Bowie L, Bagg J, et al. Risk factors for chest infection in acute stroke. Stroke 2007;38(8):2284–91.
5. Kwok C, McIntyre A, Janzen S, et al. Oral care post stroke: a scoping review. J Oral Rehabil 2015;42(1):65–74.
6. O'Malley L, Powell R, Hulme S, et al. A qualitative exploration of oral health care among stroke survivors living in the community. Health Expect 2020;23(5):1086–95.
7. Elad S, Zadik Y, Kaufman E, et al. A new management approach for dental treatment after a cerebrovascular event: a comparative retrospective study. Oral Surg Oral Med Oral Pathol Oral Radiol Endod 2010;110(2):145–50.
8. Conde-Mir I, Miranda-Rius J, Trucco E, et al. In-vivo compatibility between pacemakers and dental equipment. Eur J Oral Sci 2018;126(4):307–15.

A Child with Tetralogy of Fallot Presents for Extraction of Mandibular Premolars

Jayakumar Jayaraman, BDS, MDS, FDSRCS, MS, PhD

KEYWORDS

- Tetralogy of fallot • Cyanosis • Congenital heart disease • Children
- Dental treatment

KEY POINTS

- Children with cyanotic heart conditions are predisposed to subacute bacterial endocarditis.
- Consultation with a cardiologist is imperative before emergency and elective dental treatments.
- Anticoagulant therapy is prescribed for valvular heart disease, and children are prone to increased risk of bleeding-related complications.

A 11-year-old boy was referred for preorthodontic extractions. The patient reported a history of severe crowding in the maxillary and mandibular dentition. He has an established dental home. Clinically, he was caries free with good oral hygiene. Father reports that the child was diagnosed with tetralogy of Fallot and has undergone surgical procedure soon after birth to correct cardiac malfunction. The child is on regular cardiology follow-up, and a recent visit was unremarkable. Significant allergies include penicillin, with cutaneous rash. Current medications were warfarin (Coumadin), 5 mg, PO daily and furosemide (Lasix), 50 mg, PO daily.

On clinical examination, he was mesocephalic, with a convex profile. There was no facial asymmetry. Intraoral examination revealed permanent dentition, parabolic maxillary and mandibular arches, and angle class I molar and class II canine relationship with overjet 5 mm and overbite 70%. Severe crowding in the maxillary and mandibular anterior region and ectopic eruption of tooth #6, 11 were observed.

A panoramic was acquired to visualize the root morphology of the mandibular first premolars recommended for extraction (tooth #21, 28). Crown morphology was

Pediatric Dentistry, Children's Hospital of Richmond, Suite 200, Floor 6, 1000 East Broad Street, Richmond, VA 23219, USA
E-mail address: jayakumar83@hotmail.com
Website: http://www.rapid-statement.org

Dent Clin N Am 67 (2023) 415–417
https://doi.org/10.1016/j.cden.2023.02.008
0011-8532/23/© 2023 Elsevier Inc. All rights reserved.

normal, and roots were immature and bifurcated. Bone trabecular pattern, alveolar bone height, and lamina dura were within normal limits (**Fig. 1**).

Behavioral assessment: Frankl behavior rating scale 4 (definitely positive)—good rapport with the dentist and interest in the dental procedures.

DENTAL MANAGEMENT DECISION AND JUSTIFICATION

Initial consultation with cardiologist regarding the status of tetralogy of Fallot, history of surgery, current baseline cardiac function, medications, allergies, use of local anesthetic with epinephrine, use of nitrous oxide sedation, and the need for antibiotic prophylaxis.

Medical consultation was received from the child's cardiologist. Tetralogy of Fallot was repaired at 3 months, and the child is currently in a stable condition. He is currently taking warfarin and furosemide daily. His recent prothrombin time-international normalized ratio (PT-INR) was 2.2. There was no contraindication for the use of local anesthetic and nitrous oxide sedation. Recommended antibiotic prophylaxis 1 hour before the surgery.

Based on the consultation from the cardiologist, the child was considered for the dental procedure in the office setting. The patient was prescribed azithromycin, 500 mg, PO who took the medicine 1 hour before the start of the procedure under supervision. Considering extraction of all premolars, nitrous oxide and oxygen sedation was used at the ratio of 40:60 throughout the procedure. Following application of 20% benzocaine topical anesthesia, 4% articaine (1:100,000 epinephrine) at 7 mg/kg body weight was given as infiltration around the premolars. The gingival crestal fibers were released, and the mandibular first premolars, tooth #21, 28 were elevated and extracted using forceps. Hemostasis was achieved by placement of simple interrupted sutures using 4.0 size resorbable polyglactin (Vicryl) sutures. Postextraction instructions were given, and acetaminophen (Tylenol) was prescribed for pain, as needed. Patient was discharged on confirmation of hemostasis.

Tetralogy of Fallot is a congenital cyanotic cardiac condition characterized by ventricular septal defect, pulmonary stenosis, overriding aorta, and right ventricular hypertrophy. Surgical intervention is performed immediately after birth, and the children who are at risk of congestive heart failure are prescribed with diuretics and oral anticoagulants to prevent blood clots.[1] Children with congenital heart disease are prone for developing subacute bacterial endocarditis. Antibiotic prophylaxis is recommended for dental procedures that require manipulation of gingival tissues, including extractions. Because the child had known allergy to penicillin, as an alternate, azithromycin was prescribed. Cephalosporins should be avoided in patients with history of allergy to penicillin. The American Heart Association recently updated

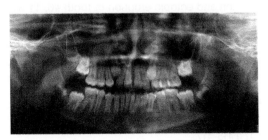

Fig. 1. Panoramic radiograph of the child showing bifurcation of roots in mandibular second premolars

its recommendation regarding clindamycin as an alternative to penicillin allergy due to community-acquired *Clostridium difficile* infection.[2] This update was adopted by the American Academy of Pediatric Dentistry.[3] Because most patients take oral anticoagulants, it is crucial to ensure that the PT-INR levels are within normal parameters, and adequate hemostasis is achieved postoperatively. Patients with congenital heart disease are prone to multitude of complications, and hence it is important to consult with the patient's cardiologist before providing oral care to these patients.

REFERENCES

1. Ansari G, Mansouri M, Eftekhar L. Dental management of a patient with pulmonary atresia and ventricular septal defect. Front Dent 2021;18:21.
2. Wilson WR, Gewitz M, Lockhart PB, et al. American heart association young hearts rheumatic fever, endocarditis and kawasaki disease committee of the council on lifelong congenital heart disease and heart health in the young; council on cardiovascular and stroke nursing; and the council on quality of care and outcomes research. prevention of viridans group streptococcal infective endocarditis: a scientific statement from the american heart association. Circulation 2021;143(20): e963–78.
3. American Academy of Pediatric Dentistry. Antibiotic prophylaxis for dental patients at risk of infection. Available at: https://www.aapd.org/globalassets/media/policies_guidelines/bp_prophylaxis.pdf. Accessed August 15, 2022.

Complete Denture Fabrication in a Patient with Chronic Obstructive Pulmonary Disease and Active Tobacco Use

Miriam R. Robbins, DDS, MS[a],*, Kimberly A. Strauch, PhD, ANP-BC[a,b]

KEYWORDS

- Complete denture • COPD • Emphysema • Supplemental oxygen • Tobacco use

KEY POINTS

- Among patients with chronic obstructive pulmonary disease (COPD), pre-procedural antimicrobial rinses, high-speed suction, and rubber dams (if tolerated) should be used to help reduce the possible inhalation of dental aerosols during procedures.
- Nitrous oxide–oxygen inhalation sedation can be used with caution in patients with mild to moderate COPD.
- Xerostomia is a common side effect of inhaled beta agonists and can lead to the increased risk of developing caries and periodontal disease.
- Inhaled corticosteroids can cause oropharyngeal candidiasis.
- Smoking cessation education is the single most important intervention for patients with COPD who use tobacco.

MEDICAL SCENARIO

A 69-year-old woman presents for fabrication of a complete upper and lower denture. She has no acute dental complaints. The patient's medical history is significant for emphysema, for which she uses 2 L of oxygen via nasal canula at night. She has a 40-pack year history of smoking cigarettes and currently smokes 10 cigarettes (one-half pack) per day. She has a chronic dry cough. She gets short of breath walking from the waiting room to the operatory. She tells you that she sleeps using three pillows. Her medications include a pro re nata (prn) albuterol inhaler, tiotropium, salmeterol/fluticasone, metoprolol, and rosuvastatin. Her blood pressure is 140/80 with a pulse of 70 beats per minute, regular rate, and rhythm. Her oxygen saturation via pulse

[a] Department of Oral Health, The University of Pennsylvania School of Dental Medicine, 240 South 40th Street, Room 209A, Philadelphia, PA 19104, USA; [b] The University of Pennsylvania School of Nursing, Claire M. Fagin Hall, 418 Curie Boulevard, Philadelphia, PA 19104, USA
* Corresponding author.
E-mail address: mrrobb@upenn.edu

Dent Clin N Am 67 (2023) 419–421
https://doi.org/10.1016/j.cden.2023.02.009
0011-8532/23/© 2023 Elsevier Inc. All rights reserved.

dental.theclinics.com

oximetry is 94% on room air, which she says is her baseline. Extraoral soft tissue examination is within normal limits. Intraoral soft tissue examination is significant for raised white patches present on the soft and hard palate and the dorsum of the posterior tongue. Her saliva appears frothy and thick and she has red fissures at the commissure of her lips bilaterally.

DENTAL MANAGEMENT DECISION AND JUSTIFICATION

Chronic obstructive pulmonary disease (COPD) refers to a group of diseases that cause persistent inflammation in the lungs, airflow obstruction (reduced expiratory outflow), and problems breathing. COPD is more commonly observed in women, individuals aged 65 and older, current and former smokers, and people with a history of asthma.[1] Primary causes of COPD include exposure to indoor or outdoor air pollutants, occupational dusts or chemicals, genetic factors (α1-antitrypsin deficiency), respiratory infections, and most commonly, first or secondhand exposure to tobacco smoke.[2]

Patients with COPD have varying degrees of compromised airway function that can affect their ability to tolerate dental treatment. Delivery of dental care may need to be altered either because of the decrease in pulmonary function or as a result of medications routinely prescribed to treat the underlying symptoms. To determine the severity and control of the patient's COPD, questions addressing exacerbating factors, frequency of signs/symptoms, and disease management protocols should be part of medical history taking. Because breathing is often compromised in a supine position (hence the patient needing three pillows to sleep), patients must often be treated sitting in a semi-Fowler's or high Fowler's position (with the head elevated in an upright position at least 30°–60° in the dental chair). Shorter appointments are also necessary if the patient cannot tolerate prolonged sitting. In patients with advanced COPD, the use of supplemental oxygen and oximetry monitoring may be necessary. Low-flow oxygen (2–3 L/min) delivered by nasal cannula should be considered if the oxygen saturation on room air is less than 92% during dental care.

The mouth is a reservoir for pathogens. Recent evidence suggests that there is a strong association between aspiration of plaque organisms and pneumonia in individuals with COPD.[3] Pre-procedural antimicrobial rinses, high-speed suction, and rubber dams (if tolerated) should be used to help reduce the possible inhalation of dental aerosols during procedures. Nitrous oxide–oxygen inhalation sedation can be used with caution in patients with mild to moderate COPD. It should not be used in patients with advanced COPD (especially emphysema) because the nitrous oxide may accumulate in air spaces of the lung potentially causing rupture of alveolar bullae.

COPD is not curable, and symptoms typically worsen over time. Medical treatment is directed at reducing the degenerative effects of the disease and providing lessening of acute symptoms. Inhaled short- and long-acting beta agonists, inhaled corticosteroids, and inhaled long-acting muscarinic antagonists are used to reduce airway inflammation and relax constricted bronchi. Xerostomia is a common side effect of inhaled beta agonists and can lead to the increased risk of developing caries and periodontal disease. Inhaled corticosteroids can cause oropharyngeal candidiasis, especially in elderly patients wearing removable prostheses or patients who are on prolonged courses of antibiotics secondary to pulmonary infections.[4] Patients should be instructed to rinse their mouths with water or use a spacer when using a corticosteroid inhaler to reduce the incidence of intraoral candidiasis. Intraoral fungal infections should be treated with either topical or systemic antifungals. Angular cheilitis can be treated with supportive measures (ie, removal and cleaning of dentures at night and application of topical emollients to the affected areas) and treated with topical antifungals and antibiotics secondary to a high incidence of coinfection with bacteria.

Smoking cessation education is the single most important intervention for patients with COPD who use tobacco. Tobacco use continues to be a major contributor to adult morbidity and mortality. A recent study reveals that approximately 45% of US adults who smoke cigarettes have received smoking-cessation advice from their dental care professionals in the past year and most patients who received smoking-cessation advice from their dental care professionals were middle-aged, reported poor health status, or had COPD.[5] Although this population may benefit greatly from tobacco cessation counseling, they are the least likely to respond to smoking-cessation advice alone and may need adjuvant therapies such as nicotine replacement therapy, pharmacologic management, intensive behavioral intervention, and psychiatric or specialist services.[5] With the proper training, dental professionals are well-positioned to play a key role in assisting patients with tobacco cessation.

DISCLOSURE

The authors have no conflicts of interest to disclose.

REFERENCES

1. Wheaton AG, Cunningham TJ, Ford ES, et al. Employment and activity limitations among adults with chronic obstructive pulmonary disease – United States, 2013. MMWR Morb Mortal Wkly Rep 2015;64(11):290–5.
2. Centers for Disease Control and Prevention. Annual smoking-attributable mortality, years of potential life lost, and productivity losses – United States, 1997–2001. MMWR Morb Mortal Wkly Rep 2005;54(250):625–8.
3. Linden GJ, Herzberg MC. Working group 4 of the joint EFP/AAP workshop. Periodontitis and systemic diseases: a record of discussions of working group 4 of the Joint EFP/AAP Workshop on Periodontitis and Systemic Diseases. J Periodontol 2013;84(Suppl 4):S20–3.
4. Devlin J. Patients with chronic obstructive pulmonary disease: management considerations for the dental team. Br Dent J 2014;217:235–7.
5. Yadav S, Lee M, Hong YR. Smoking-cessation advice from dental care professionals and its association with smoking status: analysis of the National Health and Nutrition Examination Survey 2015-2018. J Am Dent Assoc 2022;153(1): 15–22.

A Patient with a History of Extrinsic Asthma Presents for Endodontic Therapy for the Upper Molar

Miriam R. Robbins, DDS, MS[a],*, Kimberly A. Strauch, PhD, ANP-BC[b]

KEYWORDS

- Asthma • Endodontic treatment • Acute dental pain • Dental management

KEY POINTS

- Symptomatic patients presenting for emergency care should receive minimal care needed to address the urgent dental condition with follow-up treatment once asthma symptoms have resolved.
- Patients should be reminded to bring their rescue inhaler (if used) with them to all dental appointments.
- Nitrous oxide sedation is possible for patients with mild-to-moderate asthma but should be avoided in those with severe asthma.
- Potential asthma triggers during dental care should be minimized (ie, anxiety, fear, dental aerosols, and so forth).
- The use of inhaled corticosteroids can increase the risk of oral candidiasis and xerostomia.

MEDICAL SCENARIO

A 27-year-old female patient presents for an emergency visit with a chief complaint of throbbing pain on the upper right side that is unrelieved with pain medications. She has not seen a dentist in 2 years and is anxious. Examination reveals that the upper right first molar needs endodontic treatment. The patient's medical history is significant for asthma that is precipitated by dust, cat dander, and seasonal allergies. She

---

Neither author has any conflicts of interest to disclose.

Scenario 8: A patient with a history of extrinsic asthma presents for endodontic therapy of the upper molar.

[a] Department of Oral Medicine, Care Center for Persons with Disabilities, The University of Pennsylvania School of Dental Medicine, 240 South 40th Street, Philadelphia, PA 19104, USA; [b] The University of Pennsylvania School of Nursing, Claire M. Fagin Hall, 418 Curie Boulevard, Philadelphia, PA 19104, USA

* Corresponding author.

E-mail address: mrrobb@upenn.edu

https://doi.org/10.1016/j.cden.2023.02.010
dental.theclinics.com

reports that she also gets "wheezy" whenever she has a cold. Her last emergency room visit for asthma was 13 months ago, precipitated by an upper respiratory infection. She uses her rescue inhaler 2 or 3 times a week during the winter (usually after exercising) and slightly more often in the springtime. Medications include albuterol prn, fluticasone propionate, montelukast, and cetirizine. Vital signs today are 120/70 with a pulse of 92, regular rate, and rhythm. Extraoral and intraoral soft tissue examination is within normal limits.

DENTAL MANAGEMENT DECISION AND JUSTIFICATION

In the United States, 1 out of every 12 people (25 million) has a diagnosis of asthma, and the prevalence continues to increase every year.[1] Typically, asthma is a lifelong condition characterized by airway inflammation and varying degrees of expiratory airway obstruction that manifests as wheezing, shortness of breath, chest tightness, and a dry spasmodic cough that varies over time and in intensity.[2] Although several prenatal and perinatal factors have been implicated in the development of childhood asthma (ie, maternal age, smoking, diet, medication use), primary risk factors for adults with asthma include obesity, exposure to first or secondhand tobacco smoke, occupational exposures, and chronic rhinitis.[3] In addition, asthma is more common in individuals with other atopic diseases, such as atopic dermatitis and allergic rhinitis. Goals of asthma management are 2-fold: (1) to achieve good control of asthma-related symptoms and (2) to minimize the risk of future asthma exacerbations through the optimization of pharmacotherapy, minimization of environmental triggers, and prevention of recurrent exacerbations and emergency care. Pharmacological management is divided into maintenance/controller agents (inhaled corticosteroids ± long-acting β2 receptor agonists and leukotriene receptor antagonists) and rescue drugs (short-acting β2 receptor agonists and anticholinergic agents). Maintenance/controller agents are taken daily to control and prevent underlying inflammation, decrease hyperreactivity of the airway, and provide long-term bronchodilation. Rescue drugs have a rapid onset and short duration and are used to relieve acute symptoms or as a preventive measure before exposure to aggravating stimuli.

With increasing rates of asthma in the general population, dental professionals need to be able to recognize the signs and symptoms of poorly controlled asthma and modify dental treatment accordingly. The medical history and a review of systems should include information about the frequency of episodes, precipitating factors, degree of control such as rate of inhaler use, and number of episodes that required hospitalization. Patients should be reminded to bring their rescue inhaler (if used) with them to the dental appointment and to take all other medications as directed before the appointment.

A major concern in the management of asthmatic patients undergoing routine dental care is preventing an acute exacerbation. The presence of asthmatic symptoms such as wheezing, coughing, or the presence of an upper respiratory tract infection are contraindications to elective treatment, and these patients should be rescheduled. Symptomatic patients presenting for emergency care should be given the minimal care needed to address the urgent condition with plans for follow-up treatment once symptoms have resolved. A quick review of systems and confirmation that the patient has taken the most recent scheduled dose of medication should be done before initiation of emergency treatment. Anxiety is a known asthma trigger. Precipitation of an acute attack is most likely during potentially stimulating procedures such as delivery of local anesthesia, extractions, and pulpal extirpation. Nitrous oxide sedation is possible for patients with mild-to-moderate asthma but should be avoided in those with severe asthma. Patients may need to be treated with their head elevated to 45 degrees. Potential asthma triggers such as tooth and material dust and aerosolized water during drilling should be minimized. Use of a rubber dam and careful suctioning can help prevent a hyperreactive airway response.[4,5]

Common symptoms of an acute asthma exacerbation include sudden chest tightness and airflow obstruction, dyspnea with decreased expiratory volume, spasmodic coughing, inspiratory and expiratory wheezing, tachypnea, and tachycardia. As an acute episode progresses, patients often become anxious and agitated. Dental treatment should be terminated immediately. Everything should be removed from the patient's mouth, and the patient should be placed upright and allowed to assume whatever position is most comfortable (frequently patients will want to lean slightly forward). Oxygen should be administered via face mask, if available. A short-acting bronchodilator such as albuterol (a β-2 receptor agonist) should be administered and repeated every 15 minutes as needed. Corticosteroid inhalers are not appropriate for the management of an acute asthma attack.

The dental practitioner should also be aware that the use of inhaled corticosteroids can increase the risk of oral candidiasis. The oral cavity should be examined for signs and symptoms of oropharyngeal fungal infections at every visit. Patients should be instructed to use a spacer (if available) and rinse their mouth out with water immediately after inhaled corticosteroid use. The sympathomimetic agents may cause a reduction in saliva, particularly if taken in conjunction with other xerostomia-producing drugs; this may increase susceptibility to the development of dental caries. Regular dental visits and use of a preventive fluoride regimen can help reduce development of caries in this population.[6]

CLINICS CARE POINTS

- Obtain a thorough medical history, including the severity and frequency of asthma symptoms and medications used, before starting dental treatment.

- Ensure that the patient brings their inhaler to the appointment and that it is easily accessible during treatment.

- Consider using preoperative medication to help manage asthma symptoms, such as a short-acting bronchodilator or corticosteroid.

- Monitor the patient's respiratory status throughout the appointment and be prepared to stop treatment if necessary.

REFERENCES

1. Centers for Disease Control and Prevention. Vital signs: asthma in the US. Available at: https://www.cdc.gov/vitalsigns/asthma/index.html. Accessed September 27, 2022.
2. Global Initiative for Asthma (GINA). Global Strategy for Asthma Management and Prevention. Available at: www.ginasthma.org. Accessed September 27, 2022.
3. Litonjua AA, Weiss ST. Risk factors for asthma. In: Dieffenbach P, editor. UpToDate; 2022. Available at: https://www.uptodate.com/contents/risk-factors-for-asthma. Accessed September 26, 2022.

4. Robbins MR. Chapter 3: pulmonary disease. In: Patton LL, Glick M, editors. The ADA practical guide to patients with medical conditions. 2nd edition. New Jersey: Wiley-Blackwell; 2015. p. 43–69.
5. Baghani E, Ouanounou A. The dental management of the asthmatic patients. Spec Care Dentist 2021;41:309–18.
6. Maupomé G, Shulman JD, Medina-Solis CE, et al. Is there a relationship between asthma and dental caries? a critical review of the literature. J Am Dent Assoc 2010; 141(9):1061–74.

Restorative Treatment in a Patient with Chronic Obstructive Pulmonary Disease, Ischemic Heart Disease, and Arrhythmia

Kimberly A. Strauch, PhD, CRNP, ANP-BC[a,b,*],
Miriam R. Robbins, DDS, MS[a]

KEYWORDS

- COPD • Ischemic heart disease • Arrhythmia • Dental management • Restorations

KEY POINTS

- The dental environment can increase the likelihood of an anginal attack due to fear, pain, or anxiety associated with dental care.
- Patients at risk for or with known anginal symptoms should be encouraged to bring their usual antianginal therapy with them to all dental appointments.
- Local anesthetics with epinephrine should be used judiciously in patients with ischemic heart disease.
- Among patients with chronic obstructive pulmonary disease, preprocedural antimicrobial rinses, high-speed suction, and rubber dams should be used to help reduce the possible inhalation of dental aerosols during procedures.
- Patients using inhaled corticosteroids should be monitored for oropharyngeal candida.

MEDICAL SCENARIO

A 62-year-old woman presents for restorative treatment. She has no acute dental concerns. Her medical history is significant for mild chronic obstructive pulmonary disease (COPD), ischemic heart disease (IHD), and cardiac arrhythmia. The patient reports that she gets chest pain with exertion that is generally relieved with nitroglycerin and rest. She occasionally gets chest "twinges" at night that wake her from sleep. Current medications include albuterol, tiotropium bromide, budesonide/formoterol, isosorbide

[a] Department of Oral Medicine, Care Center for Persons with Disabilities, The University of Pennsylvania School of Dental Medicine, 240 South 40th Street, Philadelphia, PA 19104, USA;
[b] The University of Pennsylvania School of Nursing, Claire M. Fagin Hall, 418 Curie Boulevard, Philadelphia, PA 19104, USA
* Corresponding author.
E-mail address: kstrauch@upenn.edu

Dent Clin N Am 67 (2023) 427–430
https://doi.org/10.1016/j.cden.2023.02.011
0011-8532/23/© 2023 Elsevier Inc. All rights reserved.

dental.theclinics.com

mononitrate, amiodarone, atenolol, aspirin, and atorvastatin. Her vital signs today are 148/82 with a pulse of 84, regular rate, and rhythm. She has no known drug allergies.

DENTAL MANAGEMENT DECISION AND JUSTIFICATION

IHD and its sequelae (ie, myocardial infarction, arrhythmia, heart failure) are a common comorbidity among individuals with COPD[1] and may be more prevalent than expected beyond shared risk factors, such as aging and smoking, due to the pathophysiological effects of systemic inflammation.[2] Both conditions share common symptoms such as chest tightness or chest pain, shortness of breath at rest or with exertion, and fatigue, making it more difficult to differentiate the cause of exacerbations for either condition.

Research reveals that although IHD is a significant cause of morbidity and mortality among patients with COPD, very little is actually known about the associations of comorbid IHD with important parameters of COPD, such as symptoms in the stable and exacerbated states, health status, exercise capacity, and the frequency and severity of exacerbations.[3] What is known is that comorbid IHD is associated with overall poorer health status, lower exercise capacity, and more dyspnea in stable patients with COPD.[3]

When it comes to the dental management of patients with cooccurring IHD and COPD, it may be prudent to consult with the patient's cardiac provider to determine clinical stability for elective dental care. Individuals on QT prolonging medications such as amiodarone are at increased risk for ventricular arrhythmias and should undergo a periodic electrocardiogram for monitoring. The QT interval represents the length of time required for the heart to repolarize (relax and refill) following depolarization (contraction). The normal range for the rate-corrected QT interval (QTc) is slightly different for men and women. A QTc greater than or equal to 470 milliseconds (ms) is considered prolonged in men, and a QTc greater than or equal to 480 ms is considered prolonged in women.[4] Macrolide antibiotics should be avoided in patients with prolonged QT intervals.

Patients with a history of IHD with angina should be assessed for anginal symptoms at every dental visit. Unstable angina presents as a worsening of symptoms, onset of symptoms at lower levels of exertion, a need for increased doses of nitrates to achieve relief, or delayed/limited relief from chest pain when nitrates are used. Typically, anginal pain is precipitated by factors that increase myocardial oxygen demand, which often includes physical activity or exertion, and usually resolves with rest. Angina at rest or during sleep is considered unstable angina and should be viewed as a potential prodrome for an impending coronary event. Patients with these symptoms should be referred to their health care provider for evaluation before any dental care is initiated.[5]

Dental management of patients with stable angina includes a review of systems and vital signs before any treatment. Short appointments, usually in the morning when the patient is well rested, are preferable. An oxygen source and the patient's own nitroglycerin should be readily available in case of medical emergency. A stress reduction protocol focused on reduction of pain and anxiety may be used if indicated. Judicious use of local anesthetics with epinephrine should be used to ensure profound anesthesia and limited to no more than 0.034 mg of local anesthetic, with 1:100,000 epinephrine delivered with careful aspiration to ensure that there is no intravascular delivery.[6] Amiodarone inhibits lidocaine metabolism, increasing lidocaine serum levels and potentially causing toxicity. In this patient, articaine may be a safer alternative to reduce the possibility of toxicity.[6]

COPD is incurable and progressive over time. Medical treatment is directed at reducing the degenerative effects of the disease and providing lessening of acute symptoms. Inhaled short- and long-acting beta-agonists, inhaled corticosteroids, and inhaled long-acting muscarinic antagonists are used to reduce airway inflammation and relax constricted bronchi. Xerostomia is a common side effect of inhaled beta-agonists and can lead to an increased risk of developing caries and periodontal disease. Inhaled corticosteroids can cause oropharyngeal candidiasis, especially in elderly patients wearing removable prostheses or patients who are on prolonged courses of antibiotics secondary to pulmonary infections.[7] The candida can appear in the classic pseudomembranous form (with white curdlike patches on the surface of the oral mucosa, tongue, or palate that can be easily wiped off, leaving a raw, erythematous base) or in the erythematous form (velvety erythematous patches usually present on the palate and dorsum of the tongue). Angular cheilitis (erythematous or ulcerated fissures affecting unilaterally or bilaterally the commissures of the mouth) is an opportunistic infection of fungi and/bacteria. The incidence of intraoral candida can be reduced by having the patient use a spacer with their corticosteroid inhaler and instructing them to rinse their mouth out with water immediately after use. Intraoral fungal infections should be treated with either topical or systemic antifungals. Angular cheilitis can be treated with topical antifungal preparations with the addition of a topical antibiotic if warranted.

Because breathing is often compromised in patients with COPD if they are placed in a fully supine position, patients must often be treated with their head elevated in an upright position at 45° while in the dental chair. Shorter appointments may also be necessary depending on the patient's tolerance. There seems to be a strong association between aspiration of plaque organisms and pneumonia in individuals with COPD.[8] Having the patient rinse with an antimicrobial rinse before procedures and use of high-speed suction and rubber dams (if tolerated) can help reduce the potential inhalation of dental aerosols during procedures. In addition, patients should be encouraged to practice excellent oral hygiene, including careful daily cleaning of removable dental prostheses, to reduce the presence of plaque and biofilm in the oral cavity.

CLINICS CARE POINTS

- Patients with a history of IHD with angina should be assessed for anginal symptoms at every dental visit. This includes a review of systems to determine if the angina is stable or unstable and a complete set of vital signs before any treatment.

- Short appointments, usually in the morning, are preferable.

- An oxygen source and the patient's own nitroglycerin should be readily available in case of medical emergency.

- A stress reduction protocol focused on reduction of pain and anxiety may be used if indicated.

- Use local anesthetics with epinephrine judiciously.

- Patients who also have COPD must often be treated with their head elevated in an upright position at 45° while in the dental chair to decrease work of breathing and minimize aspiration risks.

DISCLOSURE

Neither author has any conflicts of interest to disclose.

REFERENCES

1. Soriano JB, Visick GT, Muellerova H, et al. Patterns of comorbidities in newly diagnosed COPD and asthma in primary care. Chest 2005;128(4):2099–107.
2. Sin DD, Man SFP. Why are patients with chronic obstructive pulmonary disease at increased risk of cardiovascular diseases? The potential role of systemic inflammation in chronic obstructive pulmonary disease. Circulation 2003;107(11):1514–9.
3. Patel ARC, Donaldson GC, Mackay AJ, et al. The Impact of Ischemic Heart Disease on Symptoms, Health Status, and Exacerbations in Patients with COPD. Chest 2012;141(4):851–7.
4. Berul, CI. Acquired long QT syndrome: definitions, pathophysiology, and causes. In Parikh N, editor. UpToDate; 2022. Available at: https://www.uptodate.com/contents/acquired-long-qt-syndrome-definitions-pathophysiology-and-causes. Accessed September 26, 2022.
5. Niwa H, Sato Y, Matsuura H. Safety of dental treatment in patients with previously diagnosed acute myocardial infarction or unstable angina pectoris. Oral Surg Oral Med Oral Pathol Oral Radiol Endod 2000;89(1):35–41.
6. Becker Daniel E. Cardiovascular drugs: implications for dental practice part 1-cardiotonics, diuretics, and vasodilators. Anesth Prog 2007;54(4):178–86.
7. Devlin J. Patients with chronic obstructive pulmonary disease: management considerations for the dental team. Br Dent J 2014;217:235–7.
8. Van der Maarel-Wierink CC, Vanobbergen JNO, Bronkhorst EM, et al. Oral Health Care and Aspiration Pneumonia in Frail Older People: A Systematic Literature Review. Gerodontology 2013;30(1):3–9. https://doi.org/10.1111/j.1741-2358.2012.00637.x.

An Initial Visit in a Patient with a History of Tuberculosis

Kimberly A. Strauch, PhD, CRNP, ANP-BC[a,b,*],
Miriam R. Robbins, DDS, MS[a]

KEYWORDS

- Tuberculosis • Dental management • Dental examination • Dental cleaning

KEY POINTS

- Individuals at the greatest risk of contracting tuberculosis (TB) are those with impaired immunity or those who have a higher risk of being exposed to an infection due to environmental factors.
- Individuals with active TB are highly infectious and should not receive any elective dental care until they have been deemed noninfectious.
- Individuals with active TB who require urgent dental care should be seen in a facility with a respiratory protection program and airborne infection isolation protocols.
- Individuals with latent TB infection are typically asymptomatic and noninfectious and can be treated using standard infection control protocols.

MEDICAL SCENARIO

A 35-year-old man who recently immigrated to the United States from Southeast Asia presents to the dental clinical as a new patient for an initial examination. He has no acute dental concerns. During the medical history, he states that he had a "positive" tuberculin skin test two months ago. A follow-up serum interferon-gamma release assay (IGRA) test was also positive. His chest x-ray and sputum cultures have been negative. He is currently undergoing a 4-month course of oral rifampin and vitamin B6, which were started at the time of his diagnosis. Today, his review of systems is negative and his vital signs are within normal limits.

[a] Department of Oral Medicine, Care Center for Persons with Disabilities, The University of Pennsylvania School of Dental Medicine, 240 South 40th Street, Philadelphia, PA 19104, USA;
[b] The University of Pennsylvania School of Nursing, Claire M. Fagin Hall, 418 Curie Boulevard, Philadelphia, PA 19104, USA
* Corresponding author.
E-mail address: kstrauch@upenn.edu

Dent Clin N Am 67 (2023) 431–433
https://doi.org/10.1016/j.cden.2023.02.012
0011-8532/23/© 2023 Elsevier Inc. All rights reserved.

dental.theclinics.com

DENTAL MANAGEMENT DECISION AND JUSTIFICATION

Tuberculosis (TB) is caused by the bacterium *Mycobacterium tuberculosis* and is a leading cause of death in adults worldwide.[1] *M tuberculosis* is spread via aerosolized droplets (ie, sneezing, coughing, speaking, or singing) by an infected person. Individuals at the greatest risk of contracting TB are those with impaired immunity (ie, people with HIV, taking glucocorticoids for greater than one month, solid organ or stem cell transplants, cancers, substance use disorders, malnutrition, silicosis, use of biologic medications, and chronic diseases such as diabetes, chronic obstructive pulmonary disease [COPD], and renal disease) or those who have a higher risk of being exposed to an infection due to environmental factors (ie, household contacts, birth in a TB-endemic area, and community-based settings such as hospitals, prisons, jails, nursing homes, and homeless shelters).[2] Exposure to TB can result in one of four outcomes: (1) immediate clearance of the organism; (2) primary disease or immediate onset of active disease; (3) latent (inactive) infection; or (4) reactivation of disease—onset of active disease after many years of having a latent infection. Common signs and symptoms of active TB include cough lasting greater than three weeks, hemoptysis, chest pain, lymphadenopathy, fever or chills, night sweats, fatigue, weight loss, decreased appetite, and relevant epidemiological factors as noted above.[2,3] Diagnosis of TB is based on clinical suspicion (thorough history and physical examination). Individuals meeting clinical criteria for suspected TB should have a chest radiograph *and* either a tuberculin skin test or a serum IGRA.

Individuals with primary or active TB infection will be treated according to current guidelines and counseled on home isolation precautions and respiratory etiquette. Individuals with latent TB infection (LTBI) are typically asymptomatic and noninfectious. That is, they do not feel sick, they do not have any symptoms, and they cannot spread TB to others.[3] Among individuals with LTBI and no underlying medical problems, reactivation of disease occurs in approximately 5% to 10% of cases over a lifetime.[3] The risk of reactivation is markedly increased in patients with HIV and other comorbid medical conditions.[4] Thus, reactivation of latent disease is determined by the dynamic interplay of factors attributable to both the organism and the host.

Patients with active TB can transmit the disease and should not receive any elective dental care until they have been deemed noninfectious.[5] Standard infection precautions are insufficient to prevent transmission of TB.[6] If urgent dental care is required, it should only be provided in a facility with a respiratory protection program and airborne infection isolation protocols.[7] Questions about past history of or exposure to TB as well as comorbid medical conditions that might increase the risk of active disease should be a standard part of obtaining the medical history. In addition, patients should be asked about signs and symptoms of active TB infection (persistent, productive cough for more than three weeks; hemoptysis; fever and night sweats; chest pain; and weight loss). Patients with symptoms suggestive of active TB should be given a surgical mask and immediately be referred for medical care.

Patients presenting for elective or urgent dental treatment with a history of LTBI, similar to the patient in this case, are not infectious and can be treated using standard infection control protocols. Because of the risk of reactivation, patients with LTBI are often treated proactively. Preferred treatment regimens include three months of once-weekly isoniazid plus rifapentine; four months of daily rifampin; and three months of daily isoniazid plus rifampin or six months of daily isoniazid.[8] The Centers for Disease Control and Prevention (CDC) recommends that dental office personnel receive TB training that includes the risks of transmission in dental care settings and appropriate protocols that can be used to reduce those risks.[9]

DISCLOSURE

The authors have no conflicts of interest to disclose.

REFERENCES

1. World Health Organization. Global tuberculosis report 2019. Available at: https://www.who.int/tb/publications/global_report/en/. Accessed September 23, 2022.
2. Horsburgh CR Jr. Epidemiology of tuberculosis. In: Baron EL, editor. UpToDate; 2022. Available at: https://www.uptodate.com/contents/epidemiology-of-tuberculosis. Accessed September 23, 2022.
3. Centers for Disease Control and Prevention. Tuberculosis: Basic TB Facts. Available at: http://www.cdc.gov/tb/topic/basics/risk. Accessed September 23, 2022.
4. Horsburgh CR Jr, Rubin EJ. Clinical practice. Latent tuberculosis infection in the United States. N Engl J Med 2011;364:1441.
5. Jensen PA, Lambert LA, Iademarco MF, et al. Guidelines for preventing the transmission of Mycobacterium tuberculosis in health-care settings, 2005. MMWR Recomm Rep (Morb Mortal Wkly Rep) 2005;54(RR17):1–141.
6. Occupational Safety & Health Administration. Respiratory Protection (1910.134). U.S. Department of Labor. Available at: https://www.osha.gov/pls/oshaweb/owadisp.show_document?p_id=12716&p_table=STANDARDS. Accessed September 22, 2022.
7. Cleveland JL, Robison VA, Panlilio AL. Tuberculosis epidemiology, diagnosis and infection control recommendations for dental settings: An update on the Centers for Disease Control and Prevention guidelines. J Am Dent Assoc 2009;140(9): 1092–9.
8. Sterling TR, Njie G, Zenner D, et al. Guidelines for the Treatment of Latent Tuberculosis Infection: Recommendations from the National Tuberculosis Controllers Association and CDC, 2020. MMWR Recomm Rep (Morb Mortal Wkly Rep) 2020; 69(RR1):1–11.
9. Centers for Disease Control and Prevention. Tuberculosis (TB): Infection control in health care settings. U.S. Department of Health and Human Services. Available at: https://www.cdc.gov/tb/. Accessed September 24, 2022.

Periodontal Maintenance in a Patient with a Lung Transplantation Post-COVID-19 Infection

Miriam R. Robbins, DDS, MS[a],*, Kimberly A. Strauch, PhD, ANP-BC[a,b]

KEYWORDS

- Periodontal maintenance • Lung transplant • Immunosuppression • COVID-19

KEY POINTS

- It is generally recommended that no elective dental care be performed for the first 3 to 6 months following solid organ transplantation.
- The need for antibiotic coverage before dental treatment among lung transplant patients should be made on a case-by-case basis in consultation with the patient's transplant team.
- Immunosuppressive agents can cause gingival hyperplasia, mask dental infections, cause poor or delayed healing, increase the occurrence of viral and fungal infections, and increase the risk of developing cancers of the oral cavity. Careful inspection of the oral cavity should be done at every dental visit.

MEDICAL SCENARIO

A 52-year-old man presents for periodontal maintenance. His medical history is significant for a bilateral lung transplant performed 8 months ago because of respiratory failure secondary to COVID-19 infection. Medications include mycophenolate, cyclosporine, prednisone, acyclovir, inhaled amphotericin B, and albuterol. He had been getting regular periodontal treatment every 6 months before his illness. His last dental visit was more than 2 years ago, and he reports that his gums bleed when he brushes. On examination, there is supragingival and subgingival calculus present on multiple teeth with pockets ranging from 3 to 7 mm. The treatment plan consists of 4 quadrants of deep scaling and root planing with local anesthesia and extraction of #30 secondary

[a] Department of Oral Health, Care Center for Persons with Disabilities, The University of Pennsylvania School of Dental Medicine, 240 South 40th Street, Room 209A, Philadelphia, PA 19104, USA; [b] The University of Pennsylvania School of Nursing, Claire M. Fagin Hall, 418 Curie Boulevard, Philadelphia, PA 19104, USA
* Corresponding author.
E-mail address: mrrobb@upenn.edu

Dent Clin N Am 67 (2023) 435–437
https://doi.org/10.1016/j.cden.2023.02.013
0011-8532/23/© 2023 Elsevier Inc. All rights reserved.

dental.theclinics.com

to bone loss. Vital signs today are 140/82 with a pulse of 78, regular rate and rhythm. His oxygen saturation via pulse oximetry is 97% on room air. He has no known drug allergies. He does not miss any doses of his medications.

DENTAL MANAGEMENT DECISION AND JUSTIFICATION

Early dental screening and treatment before and after solid organ transplantation are recommended infection prophylaxis measures. However, current medical guidelines are lacking, and there are no specific recommendations for dental treatment *after* lung transplantation.[1] The oral cavity contains more than 700 different strains of bacteria, which can be spread by swallowing, aspiration into the lungs, or through injuries to the oral mucosa resulting in bacteremia.[2,3] Increased amounts of bacteria in the oral cavity and periodontitis have been associated with higher rates of pneumonia, a common complication after lung transplantation.[4] Reducing plaque burden and the administration of antibiotics are 2 strategies to reduce the risk of bacteremia among posttransplant patients.[3] Despite the pathophysiological basis for these recommendations, there are no evidence-based guidelines. To date, there is only one published study focused on oral health among lung transplant patients *after* transplantation.[1] Findings from this study revealed a higher rate of current and previous caries exposure and a lower degree of caries restoration, inconsistent oral hygiene behaviors, a lack of knowledge and education about oral health recommendations such as antibiotic prophylaxis for dental care.[1]

Although evidence-based data are lacking on the impact of pretransplant dental evaluation on posttransplant infections, most transplant centers require patients to have a dental screening before solid organ transplant. Pretransplant evaluation of the patient should focus on the identification and removal of any potential sources of infection. Discussion with the patient's health-care provider should include a discussion about whether the patient is systemically stable enough to undergo dental treatment. In some cases, delaying extensive dental treatment until posttransplant is advisable. Patients who can tolerate treatment should receive care targeted at stabilizing sites of active dental disease. This may include the placement of temporary restorations or the use of chemo-mechanical agents and atraumatic restorative treatment. Potential sources of acute or chronic infection should be evaluated including partially impacted third molars and the removal of any nonrestorable teeth. Periodontal evaluation and through dental prophylaxis should be performed. Oral hygiene instruction including the importance of maintaining excellent oral health posttransplant should be reviewed.[5]

Treatment after transplantation should only be rendered after discussion with the patient's health-care provider and/or transplant surgeon to determine the patient's status. It is generally recommended that no elective dental care be performed for the first 3 to 6 months following the transplant because the patient's immune system is often significantly suppressed in the weeks to months following the transplant to prevent organ rejection.[6,7] Once the transplant patient has stabilized, they can be treated in the dental office with proper precautions. Evidence supporting the use of antibiotic coverage among patients with solid organ transplants before dental treatment is limited.[5–7] The need for antibiotic coverage before dental treatment should be made on a case-by-case basis and the patient's transplant team consulted regarding type, dose, and timing of the antibiotic. All new dental disease should be addressed, and patients should receive routine oral examinations and dental cleanings every 3 to 6 months with an emphasis on maintaining good oral health. Immunosuppressive agents can cause gingival hyperplasia, mask dental infections, cause poor or delayed healing, and increase the occurrence of viral and fungal infections. The long-term use of immunosuppressive drugs also increases the risk of developing cancers, including cancers of the oral cavity. Careful inspection of the oral cavity should be done at every dental visit. Depending on the immunosuppressive medications, it may be prudent to review a recent complete blood count with differential and comprehensive metabolic panel to ensure adequate immune, hepatic, and renal function.

CLINICS CARE POINTS

- Close communication and coordination with the patient's transplant team is essential.
- Careful inspection of the oral cavity should be done at every dental visit.
- Patients should be closely monitored during and after dental procedures for any signs of infection, such as fever, pain, or swelling.
- The importance of routone dental visits and excellent oral hygiene should be stressed.

DISCLOSURE

Neither author has any conflicts of interest to disclose.

REFERENCES

1. Marcinkowski A, Ziebolz D, Kleibrink BE, et al. Deficits in oral health behavior and oral health status in patients after lung transplantation. Clin Res J 2018;12:721–30.
2. Aas JA, Paster BJ, Stokes LN, et al. Defining the normal bacterial flora of the oral cavity. J Clin Microbiol 2005;43:5721–32.
3. Tomás I, Diz P, Tobías A, et al. Periodontal health status and bacteraemia from daily oral activities: systematic review/meta-analysis. J Clin Periodontol 2012;39: 213–28.
4. Aguilar-Guisado M, Givaldá J, Ussetti P, et al. Pneumonia after lung transplantation in the RESITRA Cohort: a multicenter prospective study. Am J Transplant 2007;7: 1989–96.
5. Lockhart PB, Loven B, Brennan MT, et al. The evidence base for the efficacy of antibiotic prophylaxis in dental practice. J Am Dent Assoc 2007;138(4):458–74.
6. Guggenheimer J, Eghtesad B, Stock DJ. Dental management of the (solid) organ transplant patient. Oral Surg Oral Med Oral Pathol Oral Radiol Endod 2003;95: 383–9.
7. Goldman KE. Dental management of patients with bone marrow and solid organ transplantation. Dental Clinics 2006;50(4):659–76.

An Adolescent with Poorly Managed Asthma Referred for Pulp Therapy in a Permanent Tooth

Jayakumar Jayaraman, BDS, MDS, FDSRCS, MS, PhD*,
Paula L. Coates, DDS, MS

KEYWORDS

- Asthma • Partial pulpotomy • Young permanent tooth • Children • Dental

KEY POINTS

- Asthma is one of the most common chronic disorders among children. Patients with uncontrolled asthma are at risk for status asthmaticus, a severe life-threatening medical emergency.
- Consultation with a pulmonologist is required before providing dental treatment.
- Medications taken for management of asthma can increase the risk of dental caries and result in immunocompromised condition including candidiasis.

MEDICAL SCENARIO

A 13-year-old male patient was referred for pulp therapy in a permanent molar.

CHIEF COMPLAINT

Pain when having hot food and cold soda.

HISTORY OF PRESENT ILLNESS

Patient noticed cavity in the lower left back tooth. Pain started 3 days back, and it aggravates on drinking cold soda and when eating hot food. Pain is short, sharp, and nonlingering.

DENTAL HISTORY

Established dental home. Visited dentist recently who noticed gross caries in lower left back tooth. The patient was referred to a pediatric dentist due to poor patient behavior.

Pediatric Dentistry, Children's Hospital of Richmond, Suite 200, Floor 6, 1000 East Broad Street, Richmond, VA 23219, USA
* Corresponding author.
E-mail address: jayakumar83@hotmail.com

Dent Clin N Am 67 (2023) 439–442
https://doi.org/10.1016/j.cden.2023.02.014
0011-8532/23/© 2023 Elsevier Inc. All rights reserved.

MEDICAL HISTORY

Mother reports that the patient was diagnosed with asthma at 5 years of age. Asthma is uncontrolled, and the patient was admitted in the emergency department 3 months back due to difficulty in breathing.

ALLERGIES

Allergies to peanuts.

MEDICATIONS

Ventolin (albuterol sulfate) inhaler as needed, Flonase (fluticasone) inhaler daily, Singulair (montelukast) inhaler daily.

CLINICAL EXAMINATION
Extraoral Examination

Unremarkable. No facial swelling or lymphadenopathy.

Intraoral Examination

Permanent dentition. Gross caries noted in the occlusal surface of the mandibular left permanent first molar, tooth #19. No pain on percussion. No intraoral swelling noted in relation to tooth #19. Tooth was responsive, and lingering pain was observed during cold testing.

Radiographic Examination

Periapical radiograph shows caries in tooth # 19 involving the enamel and dentin and extending into the distal pulp horn. Mild widening of periodontal ligament space was noted on the periapical region of the mesial and distal roots (**Fig. 1**).

Diagnosis

Dental caries in tooth #19 with reversible pulpitis.

Behavior

Frankl behavior rating scale 2 (negative)—reluctant to accept treatment, uncooperative, some evidence of negative attitude but not pronounced.

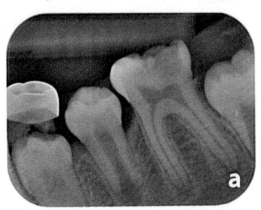

Fig. 1. Periapical radiograph showing caries in tooth #19 involving the distal pulp horn. Widening of lamina dura space is noted in the periapical region.

DENTAL MANAGEMENT DECISION AND JUSTIFICATION
Tentative Treatment Plan

Obtain consultation from a pulmonologist regarding patient's type and frequency of asthma, allergies, medications, and recommendation for management with oral conscious sedation and nitrous oxide anesthesia in the dental setting.

Medical Consultation

Medical consultation was obtained from the patient's pulmonologist indicating the patient's diagnosis of uncontrolled moderate asthma. There is a history of hospitalization 3 months back due to uncontrolled asthma, and the patient was stabilized with Albuterol nebulizer. The asthma is currently managed with Flonase and Singulair daily and Ventolin inhaler several times in a day. His recent predicted forced expiratory volume and peak flow was less than 75%. The pulmonologist had no concerns on performing dental treatment with nitrous oxide and recommended doing oral conscious sedation with a benzodiazepine. Stress dose of corticosteroid was not recommended.

Comprehensive Treatment Plan

Based on the history, clinical and radiographical evaluation, behavior of the patient, and recommendation from the pulmonologist, a partial pulpotomy and resin restoration of tooth #19 was planned with nitrous oxide and oral conscious sedation. The patient was asked to continue using the regular asthma medications at the day of surgery and asked to bring the Albuterol inhaler for use in the event of exacerbation of asthma due to stress in the dental setting. On the day of appointment, the patient was given diazepam (Valium) 0.3 mg/kg body weight 45 minutes before the procedure. Nitrous oxide to oxygen was given at 30:70 ratio; topical anesthesia and 2% lidocaine (1:100,000 epinephrine) was given as left inferior alveolar nerve block and left long buccal nerve infiltration. Rubber dam was placed, caries was excavated, and distal pulp horn coronal pulp was approached. The pulp was removed to around 2 mm depth, and hemostasis was achieved with wet sterile cotton pellet. Following application of 5.25% sodium hypochlorite on the exposed pulp, mineral trioxide aggregate partial pulpotomy was performed followed by resin-modified glass-ionomer lining and final restoration with resin restoration (**Fig. 2**). The procedure was uneventful, and Tylenol (acetaminophen) was prescribed for pain as needed. The patient was discharged under stable condition and referred to dentist for continuation of care.

Discussion

Patients with asthma have 1.5 times higher odds of the occurrence of dental caries; this is primarily due to beta-2 adrenergic agonists (Albuterol inhaler) that causes decreased salivary flow and reduction in the salivary pH.[1] In addition, patients on inhalational corticosteroids have the risk of developing opportunistic infection such as oral candidiasis, and this is attributed to immunosuppressive and antiinflammatory effects of corticosteroids.[2] It is important to use all means of behavior guidance techniques including nitrous oxide and if required, conscious sedation for anxious patients, as stress might trigger an asthmatic episode. In this patient, a benzodiazepine was recommended, as it is an anxiolytic that causes minimal respiratory depression at moderate doses. Other forms of sedation medications including meperidine or chloral hydrate are strictly contraindicated, as they could cause respiratory depression and cardiac arrest.[3] For pain control, it is recommended to use Tylenol, as other medications such as Aspirin, nonsteroidal anti-inflammatory drugs and opioids can cause histamine release, which can result in triggering an asthmatic attack.[4] Patients with

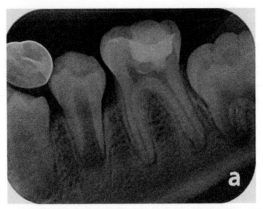

Fig. 2. Periapical radiograph showing tooth #19 treated with partial pulpotomy using mineral trioxide aggregate.

asthma can present with tendency to develop allergic reactions, and hence it is important to obtain thorough information on previous history of allergies toward food products or medicaments.

REFERENCES

1. Agostini BA, Collares KF, Costa FDS, et al. The role of asthma in caries occurrence - meta-analysis and meta-regression. J Asthma 2019;56(8):841–52.
2. Zhu JF, Hidalgo HA, Holmgreen WC, et al. Dental management of children with asthma. Pediatr Dent 1996;18(5):363–70.
3. Thomas MS, Parolia A, Kundabala M, et al. Asthma and oral health: a review. Aust Dent J 2010;55(2):128–33.
4. Chhabra K, Sood S, Sharma N, et al. Dental management of pediatric patients with bronchial asthma. Int J Clin Pediatr Dent 2021;14(5):715–8.

Adolescent Patient with Cystic Fibrosis Presents with Suspected Ludwig Angina

Jayakumar Jayaraman, BDS, MDS, FDSRCS, MS, PhD

KEYWORDS

- Cystic fibrosis • Dental abscess • Infection • Ludwig angina • Children
- Dental treatment

KEY POINTS

- Cystic fibrosis is an autosomal recessive disorder affecting multiple organs mainly respiratory and gastrointestinal organs.
- Patient's physician must be consulted before providing dental care to these patients.
- Patient with cystic fibrosis usually take broad spectrum antibiotic for prophylaxis against infections.

Patient presented with pain in the right lower back tooth region resulting in swelling of the neck.

The patient had a decayed left lower back tooth that was left unattended. Patient took acetaminophen for pain as needed. He developed pain 3 days back, which suddenly progressed into a swelling involving the face and the neck. Patient has difficulty in opening the mouth and had not eaten for the past 8 hours. He had a history of dental visit 2 years ago. The dentist noticed several dental caries and advised fillings but the patient did not follow up for treatment. Mother reports that the child was diagnosed with cystic fibrosis at 8 years. Had visited the emergency department 6 months back for acute chest infection that resolved following antibiotic medication. He denies known drug allergies. Current medications were amoxicillin with clavulanic acid 250 mg PO ter die sumendus (tds) daily, albuterol inhalation tds daily, dornase alfa, ivacaftor 150 mg PO bid daily, vitamin supplements.

On extraoral examination, the patient looked pale and febrile with dryness of lips. Bilateral swelling was noted extending into the neck below the lower border of the mandible. The lesion was hard, warm, immobile, and tender to touch (**Fig. 1**). Bilateral cervical lymph nodes were palpable and tender. He had trismus with mouth opening less than 2.5 cm. On intraoral examination, there was elevation of the tongue, grossly

Pediatric Dentistry, Children's Hospital of Richmond, Suite 200, Floor 6, 1000 East Broad Street, Richmond, VA 23219, USA
E-mail address: jayakumar83@hotmail.com

Dent Clin N Am 67 (2023) 443–446
https://doi.org/10.1016/j.cden.2023.02.015
dental.theclinics.com

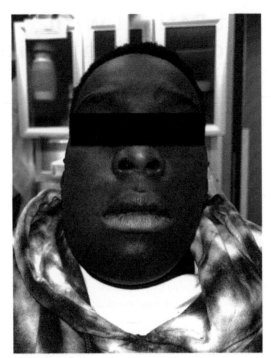

Fig. 1. Extraoral swelling involving the submandibular spaces originating from grossly carious mandibular right first permanent molar.

decayed right lower back tooth with obliteration of muco-buccal fold on the right side. Drainage was noted from the cervical margin of tooth #30 (**Fig. 2**). Periapical radiograph showed gross caries in tooth #30 with widening of lamina dura in periapical region (**Fig. 3**). Cone beam computed tomography was taken in the emergency department to visualize the extension of the dental infection.

A diagnosis of chronic caries in tooth # 30 with Ludwig angina was made.

Behavioral assessment Frankl Behavior Rating Scale 4 (Definitely Positive)—Good rapport with the dentist, interest in the dental procedures.

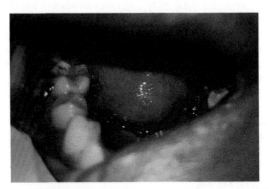

Fig. 2. Intraoral photograph showing grossly carious tooth #30 with obliteration of muco-buccal fold and drainage of abscess.

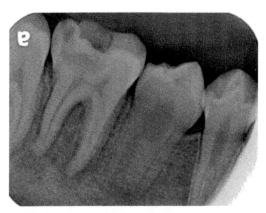

Fig. 3. Periapical radiograph showing caries involving the pulp of tooth #30 with periapical radiolucency.

DENTAL MANAGEMENT DECISION AND JUSTIFICATION

A pulmonologist was consulted to understand the status and severity of cystic fibrosis before dental management of Ludwig angina. Cystic fibrosis was diagnosed at 8 years and 6 months, and the patient is on a daily medication of amoxicillin with clavulanic acid, albuterol inhaler, dornase alfa, ivacaftor, and vitamin supplements. Based on the history, the patient was admitted to the hospital for acute chest infection 6 months back and received a dose of intravenous antibiotic therapy through indwelling central line catheter. Patient is also on a special diet along with additional pancreatic enzyme supplement. No antibiotic prophylaxis was recommended. Ampicillin with sulbactam and ibuprofen was given intravenous (IV) to control the infection and pain. The following day, the trismus was relieved, and the patient was able to open the mouth greater than 4 cm. With the help of the attending physician, ketamine was given IV for pain control. Following application of 20% benzocaine topical anesthesia, 2% lidocaine with 1:100,000 epinephrine (4.4 mg/kg) was given as right inferior alveolar nerve block and supplemented with 4% articaine with 1:100,000 epinephrine (7 mg/kg) as long buccal nerve infiltration in the right-side molar region. Tooth #30 was elevated and extracted using forceps. Hemostasis was achieved with pressure and absorbable interrupted suture with 3.0 chromic gut. Postextraction instructions were given, and the patient was monitored for another day in the hospital before discharge. Following reduction of neck swelling, the patient was able to eat solid foods, and the vital signs were found to be within normal limits. The patient was referred to the pulmonologist for follow-up and continuation of regular antibiotics for cystic fibrosis.

Patients with cystic fibrosis are prone to acquiring infection due to immunocompromised condition. This genetic disorder is caused by defective cystic fibrosis transmembrane regulator protein resulting in accumulation of fluids.[1] This condition affects multiple organs, primarily respiratory and gastrointestinal systems. Due to the risk of infection, patients are given daily prophylactic antibiotics, in addition to other supplemental medications. It is important to consult with the pulmonologist for appropriate choice of antibiotic for dental infection.[2] Because this patient was regularly taking amoxicillin with clavulanic acid, in consultation with the physician, it was decided to give ampicillin with sulbactam, a broad spectrum antibiotic through IV route. Inhalational anesthesia, including nitrous oxide is usually not indicated because patients with cystic fibrosis might develop respiratory complications. If general anesthesia is indicated, patients would require a detailed evaluation including blood gas analysis, pulmonary function test, and chest radiographs before anesthesia.[3] To relieve the source of infection, it was decided to extract the grossly carious tooth using IV ketamine to avoid complications from inhalational anesthesia. Ludwig angina of dental origin usually involves submandibular, sublingual, and submental spaces. In most cases, CBCT image is required to identify the origin and the extent of the infection. Patients require hospital admission to monitor respiratory and cardiac functions. Appropriate management with broad-spectrum antibiotic is essential to prevent the involvement of parapharyngeal and retropharyngeal spaces, which might result in mediastinitis.

REFERENCES

1. Narang A, Maguire A, Nunn JH, et al. Oral health and related factors in cystic fibrosis and other chronic respiratory disorders. Arch Dis Child 2003;88(8):702–7.
2. Fernald GW, Roberts MW, Boat TF. Cystic fibrosis: a current literature review. Pediatr Dent 1990;12(2):72–8.
3. Pawlaczyk-Kamieńska T, Borysewicz-Lewicka M, Batura-Gabryel H, et al. Oral Care Recommendation for Cystic Fibrosis Patients-Recommendation for Dentists. J Clin Med 2022;11(10):2756.

Patient Receiving Hematopoietic Stem Cell Transplantation Reports for Dental Clearance

Payam Mirfendereski, DDS[a], Katherine France, DMD, MBE[a,*]

KEYWORDS

- Hematopoietic stem cell transplantation • Dental clearance • Neutropenia
- Thrombocytopenia • Conditioning • Graft-versus-host disease

KEY POINTS

- Although no definitive consensus exists on dental treatment planning before hematopoietic stem cell transplantation (HSCT), various regimens targeted to individual patient status have been proposed.
- Oral complications during and after HSCT include oral mucositis, bleeding, opportunistic infections, hyposalivation and xerostomia, dysgeusia, nerve pain, and acute or chronic graft-versus-host disease.
- The dental provider ultimately cannot provide definitive dental clearance given the unpredictable nature of chanegs to the patient's oral and systemic status.

MEDICAL SCENARIO

A 36-year-old man presents to the dental clinic for dental clearance before planned allogeneic stem cell transplantation. His medical history is significant for recently diagnosed Philadelphia chromosome-positive acute lymphoblastic leukemia and poorly controlled depression. His most recent complete blood count demonstrates anemia (hemoglobin of 9.3 g/dL), thrombocytopenia (platelet count of 46,000/μL), and neutropenia (absolute neutrophil count of 800/μL). When asked if he has any dental complaints, he reports pain in his upper left quadrant and says he knows he has some broken teeth that need to be extracted. He mentions he has not been brushing or flossing for the past month because he does not have the motivation to care for his teeth anymore.

---

[a] Department of Oral Medicine, University of Pennsylvania School of Dental Medicine, 240 South 40th Street, Philadelphia, PA 19104, USA
* Corresponding author.
E-mail address: kfrance@upenn.edu

Dent Clin N Am 67 (2023) 447–451
https://doi.org/10.1016/j.cden.2023.02.016
0011-8532/23/© 2023 Elsevier Inc. All rights reserved.

DENTAL MANAGEMENT DECISION AND JUSTIFICATION

Dental treatment planning for the patient undergoing hematopoietic stem cell transplantation (HSCT) must be tailored to the medical status of the patient and details of planned treatment. It is a standard practice for patients planned for HSCT to obtain dental evaluation before transplant initiation given the risks associated with untreated oral infections during and after transplantation and the short-term and long-term ramifications of stem cell transplantation on the oral cavity. This assessment should be interpreted as the process of evaluating the patient's dental status and treating dental needs as appropriate to their medical status, including thorough identification of acute oral infections, dental conditions that could compromise treatment, and conditions that may progress to acute infection during the planned medical care. Dental evaluation most appropriately also includes properly educating and preparing the patient for transplantation and healing from an oral standpoint. However, the dental provider cannot provide a definitive "clearance" because they are unable to prevent the development of infection in the future or definitively predict the course of the patient's oral and systemic disease. Best efforts encompass elimination of potential sources immediate and future infections or complications.

In considering dental needs, the patient's specific medical status and urgency of transplantation will dictate the appropriate range of dental intervention. Importantly, the patient above has been referred from his oncology team for dental clearance in advance of a complex, challenging, and intensive journey, so it is paramount to communicate closely and coordinate any indicated dental treatment with the patient's oncology team.

One of the standard treatment strategies for Philadelphia chromosome-positive acute lymphoblastic leukemia (ALL), HSCT involves the infusion of stem cells from a donor to a recipient (host) to reestablish hematopoietic function.[1] Stem cell sources may include the bone marrow, peripheral blood, or umbilical cord blood. HSCTs can treat malignant and nonmalignant hematological conditions as well as certain autoimmune diseases. HSCTs can be autologous, in which the recipient is also the donor, or, as with most patients with ALL, allogeneic, in which a genetically distinct individual serves as the donor. Patients planned for HSCT undergo individualized conditioning regimens within 3 to 10 days of transplantation.[2] This conditioning regimen consists of chemotherapy with or without radiotherapy, aimed at destroying cancer cells, creating space for engraftment of donor tissue, and, in allogeneic transplant cases, achieving the immunosuppression necessary to prevent graft rejection and minimize graft-versus-host disease. The dentist should obtain relevant aspects of the timeframe and details of the HSCT plan from the patient and their oncology team before evaluation and dental treatment planning in order to appropriately tailor their care.

Although no definitive consensus exists on dental treatment planning before HSCT, the standard recommendations include the elimination of any oral foci of infection because the immunosuppressive impacts of transplant conditioning may predispose patients to bacteremia from active infectious loci and decrease the ability to withstand these changes.[2] Various protocols for dental treatment have been suggested (**Table 1**). For the patient presenting for dental assessment, it is also important to educate them on the oral complications during and after HSCT and to provide them with the tools needed to maintain their oral health throughout the treatment. Motivational interviewing can help the patient gain appreciation for and take control of their oral health. Ideal preventive care before HSCT includes oral hygiene instruction and professional dental cleaning along with fluoride treatment to minimize the oral

Table 1
Complete, partial, and minimal intervention protocols for dental treatment before hematopoietic stem cell transplantation

Protocol Type			
Dental Pathology	Complete	Partial	Minimal/Incomplete Dental Evaluation and/or Treatment Protocols/Not Cleared
Caries	Restore all teeth	Mild/moderate caries were restored if time permitted; otherwise, these lesions were left alone and observed	Intervention only if symptomatic
Severe caries/pulp involvement/dental abscess	Root canal treatment or extract		
Apical periodontitis	• Retreat • Apicoectomy • Extract	• Symptomatic lesions and lesions ≥5 mm were treated • Asymptomatic lesions and lesions <5 mm were observed	
Advanced periodontal disease	Extract teeth with • Probing depth ≥ 6 mm • Furcation I, II, III	Extract teeth with • Probing depth ≥ 8 mm • Mobility III • Severe inflammation	
Mobile primary teeth	Extract teeth with >50% root resorption	Extract teeth with severe mobility and expected to exfoliate within a few weeks	
Partially erupted third molars	Extract	• Asymptomatic teeth were observed • Partially erupted third molars with purulence of pericoronitis were extracted	

Reprinted with permission from Hong CHL, Hu S, Haverman T, et al. A systematic review of dental disease management in cancer patients. Support Care Cancer. 2018;26(1):155-174.

microbial load and caries risk before treatment and minimize accumulation of natural oral flora during and after HSCT. Chlorhexidine gluconate 0.12% rinse can be prescribed to further decrease the microbial load and reduce the risk of infection.[3] Complications during the conditioning regimen include oral mucositis, bleeding, opportunistic infections, hyposalivation and xerostomia, and dysgeusia. Effective oral hygiene can reduce the incidence of many of these complications.[2] Acute or chronic graft-versus-host disease is a common complication of allogeneic HSCT that can affect the oral cavity and complicate the patient's ongoing dental status, including through generalized inflammation, discomfort, difficulties with nutrition, and other consequences that may present challenges to maintaining hygiene and function depending on the manifestation and extent.

Dental treatment before HSCT should be aimed at controlling dental caries and periodontal disease as much as feasible. It is equally important to take measures to minimize potential sources of soft tissue trauma, given the risk for delayed healing after chemotherapy or radiotherapy. Invasive dental procedures, including extraction of hopeless teeth, can be considered in accordance with the patient's hematological status and timeframe of the HSCT.[4] If invasive treatments are to be performed, it is recommended that they be completed at least 2 weeks before the start of the conditioning regimen to allow sufficient time for soft tissue healing.[2,5] The hematological status of the patient will inform any necessary precautions. It is recommended that patients with an absolute neutrophil count less than $500/\mu L$ receive antibiotic prophylaxis before invasive dental treatment if the procedure cannot be deferred, whereas prophylaxis may be considered in accordance with other patient factors in patients with neutrophil counts between 500 and $1000/\mu L$.[2] Local hemostatic measures may be sufficient in patients with platelet counts as low as $50,000/\mu L$.[2] Platelet transfusions should be considered preoperatively and postoperatively in case of an invasive procedure planned for a patient with a platelet count at or less than $30,000/\mu L$.[6] Again, coordination with the patient's oncology team is important before proceeding with any invasive dental treatment.

CONFLICT OF INTEREST

All authors declare that they have no commercial or financial conflict of interest related to the material in this article and have received no funding for the preparation of this article.

REFERENCES

1. DeFilipp Z, Advani AS, Bachanova V, et al. Hematopoietic Cell Transplantation in the Treatment of Adult Acute Lymphoblastic Leukemia: Updated 2019 Evidence-Based Review from the American Society for Transplantation and Cellular Therapy. Biol Blood Marrow Transplant 2019;25(11):2113–23.
2. Samim F, Ten Böhmer KL, Koppelmans RGA, et al. Oral Care for Hematopoietic Stem Cell Transplantation Patients: A Narrative Review. Oral Health Prev Dent 2019;17(5):413–23.
3. Bollero P, Passarelli PC, D'Addona A, et al. Oral management of adult patients undergoing hematopoietic stem cell transplantation. Eur Rev Med Pharmacol Sci 2018;22(4):876–87.
4. Hong CHL, Hu S, Haverman T, et al. A systematic review of dental disease management in cancer patients. Support Care Cancer 2018;26(1):155–74.
5. Elad S, Raber-Durlacher JE, Brennan MT, et al. Basic oral care for hematology-oncology patients and hematopoietic stem cell transplantation recipients: a

position paper from the joint task force of the Multinational Association of Support-ive Care in Cancer/International Society of Oral Oncology (MASCC/ISOO) and the European Society for Blood and Marrow Transplantation (EBMT). Support Care Cancer 2015;23(1):223–36.

6. Bogusławska-Kapała A, Hałaburda K, Rusyan E, et al. Oral health of adult patients undergoing hematopoietic cell transplantation. Pre-transplant assessment and care. Ann Hematol 2017;96(7):1135–45.

Dental Management of the Human Papilloma Virus-Related Oropharyngeal Cancer Patient

Jillian Rigert, DMD, MD[a,*], Andres Pinto, DMD, MPH, MBA, MSCE[b],
Mel Mupparapu, DMD, MDS, Dipl.ABOMR[c]

KEYWORDS

- Radiation therapy • Head and neck cancer • Osteoradionecrosis

KEY POINTS

- Radiation therapy to the head and neck leads to lifelong risks and changes to patients' oral health.
- The radiation oncology and dental teams must collaborate before and after radiation therapy to optimize patient outcomes.
- The prevention of radiation toxicity to normal tissues is preferred when possible.
- The optimization of patient oral health status and oral hygiene is key in prevention of long-term radiation-associated orofacial sequelae.
- Limitations in current prevention and treatment options for radiation-associated orofacial sequelae demand for additional research.

A 46-year-old man with newly diagnosed human papilloma virus (HPV) + oropharyngeal cancer (OPC) was referred from radiation oncology for a pre-radiation dental examination and treatment.

The review of the radiation oncology referral reveals that patient has been diagnosed with early stage, T1N0M0 right base of tongue HPV + OPC.[1] He will be treated with radiation with curative intent. The review of medical history reveals no other medical diagnoses. Patient denies the use of alcohol, tobacco, or illicit drugs. Patient reports irregular dental visits and does not have an established dentist. He reports intermittent pain in the lower right quadrant that sometimes wakes him up at night. No history of swelling or pain on biting. Patient's goals are to maintain dentition. He feels motivated to improve oral hygiene and commit to regular dental follow-ups postradiation.

[a] Department of Radiation Oncology, University of Texas MD Anderson Cancer Center, 1515 Holcombe Boulevard, Houston, TX 77030, USA; [b] Case Western Reserve University School of Dental Medicine, Oral and Maxillofacial Medicine and Diagnostic Science, 10900 Euclid Avenue, Cleveland OH 44106-734, USA; [c] Department of Oral Medicine, University of Pennsylvania School of Dental Medicine, 240 South 40th Street, Philadelphia, PA 19104-6030, USA
* Corresponding author.
E-mail address: JMRigert@MDAnderson.org

Dent Clin N Am 67 (2023) 453–456
https://doi.org/10.1016/j.cden.2023.02.017
0011-8532/23/© 2023 Elsevier Inc. All rights reserved.

DENTAL MANAGEMENT DECISION AND JUSTIFICATION

A comprehensive extraoral and intraoral head and neck examination and dental examination with periodontal probing, charting of dental conditions and panoramic x-rays, bitewings, and periapical x-rays are completed.[2]

Patient has 28 teeth and a history of third molar extractions. Class II amalgam restorations are present on teeth #14, 19, and 30. Class II composite restorations are present on teeth #5 and 12. Tooth #30 presents with large recurrent decay extending toward pulp. Following the application of Endo-Ice on tooth #30, the patient experienced pain which lingered following removal of the Endo-Ice. He experienced mild discomfort on percussion andno pain on palpation around tooth #30. Probing depths throughout the mouth are 2 to 3 mm with mild bleeding on probing. Oral hygiene is fair with generalized plaque accumulation and moderate localized calculus build up on the lingual of the mandibular anterior dentition. No oral lesions visible in the oral cavity.

Panoramic and full mouth radiographs are obtained. Radiographically, there was no evidence of osseous changes, with the exception of apical radiolucencies around mesial and distal roots of tooth #30.

In the setting of clinical and radiographic examination findings, tooth #30 is diagnosed with irreversible pulpitis and chronic apical periodontitis.

Dental treatment plan is established to include dental cleaning and options for root canal therapy, core build-up, and crown or extraction of tooth #30 due to the extent of decay and lifetime risk of osteoradionecrosis (ORN) post-radiation.[2–4] ORN risk is elevated due to predicted radiation to the area of tooth #30 to be greater than 60 Gy per radiation oncology treatment plan.[2] Patient is counseled on treatment options and risks,[2–4] and he elects to save the tooth.

The dental cleaning and root canal therapy of tooth #30 is completed as soon as possible following the initial pre-radiation examination, and tooth #30 is restored with a nonmetallic restoration to reduce radiation scatter associated with metallic restorations with plan to return for the definitive crown after radiation therapy to reduce delays in radiation start.

Following restoration of tooth #30, an oral radiation stent is created for the patient to use during radiation therapy per the radiation oncology team, designed to displace normal tissues out of the radiation beam path and assist with positioning the patient in a repeatable position so that the radiation delivery is predictable.[5]

Owing to the risk for radiation caries in the setting of radiation exposure and anticipated salivary gland hypofunction,[3] the patient is counseled on the recommendation for prescription fluoride trays and brush on fluoride toothpaste, with improved contact time of fluoride with the use of trays. He elected to proceed with fabrication of fluoride trays, voicing understanding that a new mandibular tray will likely be needed following definitive crown restoration of tooth #30. He was prescribed fluoride gels and brush on prescription fluoride toothpaste.

Patient is counseled on the risk of lifelong radiation-attributable orofacial side effects, including salivary gland hyposalivation, xerostomia, radiation caries, trismus, dysphagia, and osteoradionecrosis.[2,3] He is advised to follow-up with the dental team at increased frequency starting with every 3 months post-radiation due to anticipated radiation-attributable oral changes, targeting early identification and intervention of issues.

Patient education hand-outs provided for reference to above information, and office number provided for questions and follow-up.

HIGHLIGHTS AND ADDITIONAL CONSIDERATIONS

- HPV (+) head and neck cancers often impact patients at younger ages with less medical compromise and are associated with more favorable prognoses compared with HPV (−) HNC counterparts. HPV (+) cancers are often radiosensitive; however, radiation is associated with acute and chronic oral health side effects that may compromise patient quality of life post-cancer treatment.[1,2]
- Cancer treatment requires multidisciplinary treatment and collaboration. Dentists are important members of the multidisciplinary treatment team. Owing to the challenges and limitations in treatment of radiation-attributable oral health sequelae, prevention of toxicities and early intervention are key.[2–5]
- The patient was provided the option for extraction of tooth #30. Pre-radiation and post-radiation extractions have been associated with the development of osteoadionecrosis, especially in the posterior mandible. If the patient was to elect for extraction of the tooth, the extraction should be performed 2 to 3 weeks pre-radiation start date to allow for soft tissue healing.
- The patient is closely monitored prior, during, and after radiation. Dental follow-up occurs at increased frequency post-radiation with common recommendation for every 3 months to identify issues early.
- If future extractions need to occur, optimize perioperative management to reduce risk for osteoradionecrosis (ORN). Current management considerations include perioperative hyperbaric oxygen (HBO) versus pentoxifylline and vitamin E.[4] More research is needed to understand efficacy of these treatment modalities and their risks versus benefits for each patient.
- Treatment recommendations for ORN remain controversial and include conservative measures (ie, oral hygiene optimization, chlorhexidine, saline rinses, and antibiotics), surgery, HBO, and/or pentoxifylline and vitamin E.[4] More research is needed to understand efficacy of these treatment modalities and their risks versus benefits for each patient. As this research is evolving, review evidence and protocol updates to inform your clinical decisions. ORN often warrants referral to oral and maxillofacial surgery for specialist management.

CLINICS CARE POINTS

- A comprehensive dental examination and optimization of oral health status should be completed for all patients with head and neck cancer prior to radiation treatment.
- Radiation therapy results in normal tissue toxicity and lifetime risk of chronic orofacial sequelae including hyposalivation and xerostomia (dry mouth), radiation caries, trismus, and osteoradionecrosis.
- Prevention of radiation toxicities and orofacial sequelae is key. The dentist has an important role in educating patients about their oral health risks and supporting patients in reducing risks through good oral hygiene, nutrition, social behaviors, routine dental follow-ups, early detection and intervention of any dental disease and oral pathology.

DISCLOSURE

J. Rigert receives salary support from the NIDCR, United States Supplement Grant 3R01DE028290-02S1.

REFERENCES

1. Economopoulou P, Kotsantis I, Psyrri A. Special issue about head and neck cancers: HPV positive cancers. Int J Mol Sci 2020;21(9):3388.
2. Yong CW, Robinson A, Hong C. Dental evaluation prior to cancer therapy. Front Oral Health 2022;3:876941.
3. Sroussi HY, Epstein JB, Bensadoun RJ, et al. Common oral complications of head and neck cancer radiation therapy: mucositis, infections, saliva change, fibrosis, sensory dysfunctions, dental caries, periodontal disease, and osteoradionecrosis. Cancer Med 2017;6(12):2918–31.
4. Lajolo C, Rupe C, Gioco G, et al. Osteoradionecrosis of the jaws due to teeth extractions during and after radiotherapy: a systematic review. Cancers 2021;13(22): 5798.
5. Stieb S, Perez-Martinez I, Mohamed ASR, et al. The impact of tongue-deviating and tongue-depressing oral stents on long-term radiation-associated symptoms in oropharyngeal cancer survivors. Clin Transl Radiat Oncol 2020;24:71–8.

An Adolescent Patient Reports to Dental Office for Pain in Relation to Mandibular Molar with an Incidental Palpable Thrill in the Submandibular Region

Leonard Jensen, DMD[a], Andres Davila, DMD[a],
Andres Pinto, DMD, MPH, MBA, MSCE, Dipl.ABOM[b],
Mel Mupparapu, DMD, MDS, Dipl.ABOMR[a],*

KEYWORDS

- Necrotic pulp • Symptomatic apical periodontitis • Thrill • Bruit
- Arteriovenous malformation • Vascular malformation

KEY POINTS

- Thorough evaluation is necessitated when encountering an atypical clinical finding associated with an endodontically involved molar.
- If an arteriovenous malformation (AVM) of the oral cavity is suspected, a triad of tooth mobility, gingival bleeding, and a radiographic finding revealing a radiolucent area are commonplace.
- AVMs of the head and neck area may be a life-threatening entity. Therefore, before initiating invasive dental treatment, interdisciplinary assessment and management of the AVM with vascular surgery are recommended to determine the best course of treatment.

MEDICAL SCENARIO

A 20-year-old female patient with a noncontributory medical history presents to the dental clinic with a chief complaint of pain in the mandibular left posterior area of 1 week duration. The patient was not on any medications other than ibuprofen and

[a] Department of Oral Medicine, University of Pennsylvania School of Dental Medicine, 240 South 40th Street, Philadelphia, PA 19104, USA; [b] Department of Oral & Maxillofacial Medicine & Diagnostic Sciences, Case Western Reserve University, 10900 Euclid Avenue, Cleveland, OH 44106, USA
* Corresponding author.
E-mail address: mmd@upenn.edu

Dent Clin N Am 67 (2023) 457–459
https://doi.org/10.1016/j.cden.2023.02.018
0011-8532/23/© 2023 Elsevier Inc. All rights reserved.

has no known drug allergies. A head and neck examination revealed a non-tender, warm, swelling in the left submandibular area with a palpable thrill and a bruit heard on auscultation. Intraoral examination revealed deep occlusal caries on a rotated tooth 19 (mandibular left first molar) tested non-vital. A periapical radiograph revealed gross carious lesion, and a diffuse periapical radiolucency was noted in relation to tooth 19. Moderate swelling was noted in the left buccal sulcus. Localized gingival bleeding in the area of tooth 19 was present, but no abnormal probing depths or sinus tracts were noted. Tooth 19 was mobile.

DENTAL MANAGEMENT DECISION AND JUSTIFICATION

Patients presenting to dental clinics for treatment of pain and swelling are common in dentistry. Most of these patients have infections related to periodontal disease and/or endodontically involved teeth, and the treatment options are variable. Most dentists would not usually consider an arteriovenous malformation (AVM) to be the cause of swelling, particularly if the swelling appears in the vicinity of a non-vital tooth or a periodontal abscess. The unique characteristics of this lesion, thrill and bruit, should alert the clinician to the unusual and very concerning nature of the swelling.

AVMs are predominantly high-flow vascular malformations with a male:female ratio of 1:2.[1] The etiology and pathogenesis of AVMs remain undefined. The proposed pathogenesis includes disturbance in vascular development during embryogenesis, potential involvement in vascular endothelial growth factor and platelet-derived growth factor, and genetic involvement such as mutations in the tumor growth factor-beta signaling pathway and the second-hit hypothesis.[1,2]

AVMs of the head and neck area are rare and may be found in hard or soft tissues. They may present in multiple sites of the oral cavity, the most common location being the anterior two-thirds of the tongue.[1,3] If present in the oral cavity, a triad of tooth mobility, gingival bleeding, and a radiographic finding revealing a radiolucent area are commonplace.[1,3] Additional clinical manifestations of hard tissue AVMs involving the oral cavity may include root resorption, tooth displacement, and bone expansion leading to physical asymmetry.[1,3] Soft tissue AVMs typically present as slow-growing masses with a port-wine hue of the overlying tissue commonly appreciated in the first or second decade.[1] On evaluation of the pulsatile lesion, vascular thrills can be identified with palpable vibrations, auscultation, and localized hyperthermia of the overlying area.[1]

Multi-imaging modalities are recommended for the diagnosis of AVMs. Gold standard imaging for diagnosing AVMs is color duplex ultrasonography.[1] Computed tomography and MRI may help determine the extent of involvement and tumor exclusion.[4] AVMs may also present in panoramic radiographs as multilocular radiolucencies with a honeycomb or soap bubble appearance.[1] The astute clinician should confirm radiographic findings with clinical presentations to avoid misinterpreting for ameloblastoma, odontogenic keratocyst, or other lesions of similar radiographic presentation.

AVMs of the head and neck may be a life-threatening entity. Most AVMs are diagnosed in the setting of hemorrhage and in the oral cavity may present as a potential, life-threatening hemorrhage revealed after surgical intervention.[1] Therefore, before initiating invasive treatment, interdisciplinary assessment and management of the AVM with vascular surgery are recommended to determine the best course of treatment.[1,4] To date, no specific antibiotic prophylaxis protocol in the oral AVMs setting exists. However, measures to prevent bacteremia during treatment are recommended to reduce the risk of infection.[1]

Based on the clinical and radiographic findings, a diagnosis was made of symptomatic apical periodontitis secondary to dental caries in the setting of a possible vascular

pathology. Treatment options were given to the patient that included either an end-odontic therapy or an extraction but not before a referral to a vascular or a head and neck surgeon to investigate further and treat the AV malformation. Definitive treatment for AVM depends on the site and is treated via surgery. Choosing endovascular embolization or stereotactic radiosurgery is the common treatment modalities used to treat AVM. Additional treatment modalities for intraosseous AVMs include osseous curettage, bone resection with reconstruction, and antiangiogenic therapy.[5] Dental treatment without a proper diagnosis of the AVM or failure to notice or take action to treat AVM will lead to uncontrolled bleeding and may result in fatal incidents.

SUMMARY

A young female patient presents to a dental clinic for treatment of swelling and pain. Clinical examination and testing are completed revealing concomitant, suspected vascular pathology of the head and neck area. An endodontic diagnosis is made, but an unusual clinical finding of a vascular entity, not typically considered by dentists, requires interdisciplinary assessment and management with vascular surgery before surgical intervention of the oral cavity.

CLINICS CARE POINTS

- Any lesion with a palpable thrill needs to be investigated to rule out an AVM before a dental procedure as AVM can be a life threatening entity if undiagnosed and untreated.
- Color duplex ultrasonography is the gold standard imaging but other imaging modalities like CT/MR may be helpful in defining the extent of the lesion.
- Dental panoramic radiographs may show an AVM as a multilocular radiolucency with a honey comb or soap bubble appearance.

DISCLOSURE

None.

REFERENCES

1. Chawla A, Gill S, Sharma S, et al. Endodontic implications of a patient with arteriovenous malformation: a case report and literature review. Int Endod J 2021;54(6): 975–87.
2. Fernández-Alvarez V, Suárez C, de Bree R, et al. Management of extracranial arteriovenous malformations of the head and neck. Auris Nasus Larynx 2020;47(2): 181–90.
3. Blackhall KK, Ling E, Kunjur J. A rare case of a intraosseous arteriovenous malformation of the temporomandibular joint and mandible - Case report and literature review. Int J Surg Case Rep 2020;76:394–8.
4. Abdel Razek AAK, Elmokadem AH, Soliman M, et al. MR Imaging of vascular malformations and tumors of head and neck. Magn Reson Imaging Clin N Am 2022; 30(1):199–213.
5. Ciccarese F, Chauvel-Picard J, Guibaud L, et al. Management of intra-osseous arteriovenous malformations of the mandible. J Stomatol Oral Maxillofac Surg 2022;123(5):e544–8.

Mönckeberg Medial Arteriosclerosis in a Geriatric Patient with Chronic Kidney Disease and Poorly Controlled Diabetes Reporting for a Dental Recall Visit

Leonard Jensen, DMD[a],*, Ali Z. Syed, BDS, MHA, MS, Dipl. ABOMR[b],
Scott Odell, DMD[a], Karoline E. Genung, RDH, BS, PHDHP[a],
Mel Mupparapu, DMD, MDS, Dipl. ABOMR[a]

KEYWORDS

- Diabetes • Chronic kidney disease • Medial arterial calcinosis • Rail-tracking
- Mönckeberg medial arteriosclerosis

KEY POINTS

- Cardiovascular disease is the leading cause of death worldwide with several comorbid etiologic factors.
- Calcification within the tunica media layer of the arteries is termed medial arterial calcification or Mönckeberg medial arteriosclerosis and is commonly noted in patients with long-standing diabetes and chronic kidney disease.
- Radiographically, the calcifications appear as "tram-tracking" or "pipe-stem" vessels that are diagnostic indicators for this condition.
- Because this condition results in compromised blood flow to the extremities, prompt recognition and treatment are beneficial to the patient.

MEDICAL SCENARIO

A 69-year-old man presents to the dental clinic for a routine recall examination. A review of the medical history revealed that the patient is a type 2 diabetic of long-standing history, suffers from stage 4 chronic kidney disease, and is on hemodialysis

[a] University of Pennsylvania School of Dental Medicine, 240 South 40th Street, Philadelphia, PA 19104, USA; [b] Case Western University School of Dental Medicine, 9601 Chester Avenue, Cleveland, OH 44106, USA
* Corresponding author.
E-mail address: leonardj@upenn.edu

Dent Clin N Am 67 (2023) 461–464
https://doi.org/10.1016/j.cden.2023.02.019
0011-8532/23/© 2023 Elsevier Inc. All rights reserved.

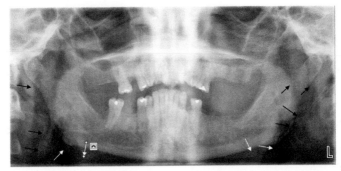

Fig. 1. Panoramic radiograph of the patient showing the pipe-stem or tram-tracking calcifications known to be from the medial arterial calcification. Branches of external carotid are well demarcated (*black arrows*). Note calcification within facial arteries bilaterally (*white arrows*).

(**Figs. 1** and **2**). Other comorbidities are hypertension, hyperlipidemia, and benign prostatic hyperplasia (BPH). His point-of-care blood glucose was 426 mg/dL. During this visit, a panoramic radiograph was obtained. Upon reviewing the panoramic radiograph, a tortuous tram-tracking was seen bilaterally in the submandibular areas proceeding superiorly with branching to include various vessels of the head and neck.

DENTAL MANAGEMENT DECISION AND JUSTIFICATION

Worldwide, cardiovascular disease is the leading cause of the death. Globally, in 2017, 17 million deaths were reported owing to cardiovascular disease. Deaths amounting to

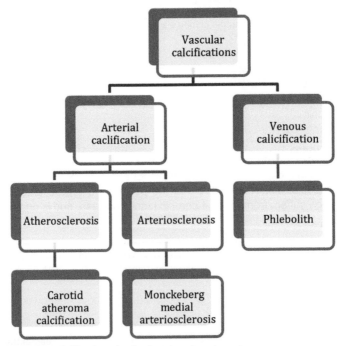

Fig. 2. The vascular calcifications in the head and neck region.

6.17 million were reported because of stroke.[1] Vascular calcifications are broadly classified into arterial and venous calcifications. Arterial calcifications are referred to in the literature by different names, such as Mönckeberg medial arteriosclerosis (MMA) and medial arterial calcification. MMA results from a calcification of the tunica media in vessels and is commonly seen in diabetic patients and those with chronic kidney disease and is usually discovered incidentally on imaging the oral and maxillofacial regions.[2] Radiographically, they appear as tram-tracking or "pipe-stem" vessels. This was first described in 1903 by Mönckeberg. This is not to be confused with atherosclerosis, which affects the tunica intima of vessels. It is now thought to be driven by hyperphosphatemia.[1,2] MMA is noted in certain disease conditions, such as diabetes, hyperparathyroidism, hypervitaminosis D, chronic kidney disease, and in patients on hemodialysis. Usually, MMA is not seen patients younger than 50 years.

It is important to note that this patient is suffering from both poorly controlled diabetes and chronic kidney disease.[2,3] MMA in major vessels puts the patient at significant risk of adverse cardiovascular outcomes owing to reduced elasticity of vessels that can result in compromised blood flow to the extremities. The importance of recognizing the radiographic appearance of this condition lies in alerting the clinician to the presence of potentially serious underlying systemic disease.[4,5] Management of MMA primarily depends on the identification of its associated conditions. Avoiding antibiotics and analgesics that are metabolized in the kidneys is a key factor in the management of these patients. Review of comorbid cardiac, renal, and endocrine issues should be attended to before a dental treatment is initiated.

MMA is usually asymptomatic and often noted as an incidental finding on imaging.[5] Hence, the appropriate knowledge about radiographic features, often subtle, may assist the clinician in the diagnosis and management of the patient.

CLINICS CARE POINTS

- Medial arterial calcification (MAC) or Mönckeberg Medial Arteriosclerosis (MMA) appears radiographically as "tram-tracks" and is noted mostly as an incidental finding on imaging.
- MAC or MMA is not seen in patients younger than 50. It is commonly associated with Diabetes, Hyperparathyroidism, Hypervitaminisos D, Chronic kidney disease, and in patients on hemodialysis.
- When the tram tracks are noted on radiographs, they alert the clinician to the presence of an underlying serious systemic condition and hence should be referred back to the appropriate medical specialist for treatment.

DISCLOSURE

The authors have nothing to disclose.

REFERENCES

1. Dos Santos VP, Pozzan G, Castelli V, et al. Arteriosclerosis, atherosclerosis, arteriolosclerosis, and Monckeberg medial calcific sclerosis: what is the difference? J Vasc Bras 2021;20:e20200211.
2. Syed AZ, Xu Y, Alluri LS, et al. Mönckeberg's Medial Arteriosclerosis in the Oral and Maxillofacial Region: A Pilot Study. Oral Dis 2022. https://doi.org/10.1111/odi.14393. Accepted Author Manuscript.

3. Shahid K, Weng S, Cook L, et al. Detection of Monckeberg Medial Sclerosis on Conventional Dental Imaging. J Mich Dent Assoc 2017;99(3):40–2, 68-69.

4. Omami G. Monckeberg Arteriosclerosis: A Telltale Sign. J Oral Maxillofac Surg 2017;75(11):2383–4.

5. Tahmasbi-Arashlow M, Barghan S, Kashtwari D, et al. Radiographic manifestations of Mönckeberg arteriosclerosis in the head and neck region. Imaging Sci Dent 2016;46(1):53–6.

Patient with Hemophilia A Presenting for Extractions and Implants

Temitope T. Omolehinwa, BDS, DMD, DScD*,
Adeyinka Dayo, BDS, DMD, MS

KEYWORDS

- Hemophilia A • Bleeding disorders • Factor VIII deficiency
- Dental management of bleeding disorders • Coagulation bleeding disorders

KEY POINTS

- Dental management of patients with Hemophilia A requires consult with the treating hematologist.
- Life-threatening bleeding can occur depending on the severity of hemophilia A, if management protocols are not followed.
- Managing patients with hemophilia A requires patient-specific treatment plans.

MEDICAL SCENARIO

A 57-year-old Caucasian male patient presented to the dental clinic for consult for implant placement as well as comprehensive oral health care. He has a history of hereditary hemophilia A and has had multiple hospitalizations from bleeding complications. There were no positive findings on the review of systems. He reports a family history of Hemophilia A in his dad and brother.

On examination, we noted multiple restorations, root-treated teeth, and missing teeth. Intraoral periapical radiographs revealed subgingival calculus as well as carious lesion on mesial of upper left first premolar (tooth #12) and periapical radiolucency on lower left first premolar and lower left lateral incisor (teeth #21 and #23), with widening of the lamina dura around #23 as well as severe bone loss (**Fig. 1**).

DENTAL MANAGEMENT DECISION AND JUSTIFICATION

The treatment plan for the above patient included scaling and root planning in all four quadrants due to the presence of subgingival calculus, extractions of #21 and #23 and

Department of Oral Medicine, Penn Dental Medicine, University of Pennsylvania, Room 212 Schattner Building, 240 South 40th Street, Philadelphia, PA 19104, USA
* Corresponding author.
E-mail address: omote@upenn.edu

Dent Clin N Am 67 (2023) 465–468
https://doi.org/10.1016/j.cden.2023.02.020
0011-8532/23/© 2023 Elsevier Inc. All rights reserved.

dental.theclinics.com

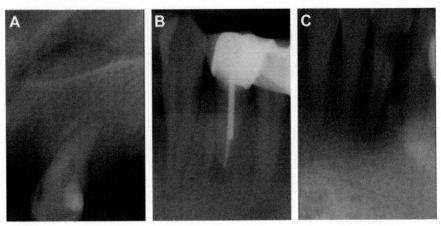

Fig. 1. (*A*) Intraoral periapical radiograph of #12 showing caries mesial of #12. (*B*) Intraoral periapical radiograph of #21 showing periapical radiolucency at the apex of an endodontically treated and crowned tooth. (*C*) Intraoral periapical radiograph of #23 showing subgingival calculus vertical bone loss distal of #23, extensive caries extending from the enamel to the pulp distally and periapical radiolucency at the apex of the same tooth.

composite restoration on #12. All procedures require tissue manipulation, with inclusion of the tooth restoration (a premolar band and wedge would have to be placed around #12 to restore the tooth's anatomy). Bleeding disorders most often require consult with hematology before treating patient. We also discussed the replacement options for the missing teeth including, implants versus bridge versus dentures versus doing nothing. We cleared the patient for noninvasive treatment only at this time and sent a consult out to the hematologist, as is standard practice before commencing invasive dental treatment in patients with hemophilia. The consult request included:

1. Hemophilia staging
2. Management protocol specific to the patient for invasive dental treatment

Consult request return, showed that patient has moderate hemophilia A, with.

a. prolonged activated partial thromboplastin time
b. normal prothrombin time
c. Factor VIII deficiency

The patient-specific treatment management protocol recommended by the hematologist is as seen below. This is especially true for procedures requiring tissue manipulation including extractions and scaling and root planning.

Preprocedure treatment:

1. Tranexamic acid 1300 mg orally every 8 hours the evening before procedure
2. Recombinant factor VIII 50 units/kg (intravenous [IV])

POSTPROCEDURE TREATMENT

1. Tranexamic acid 1300 mg orally every 8 hours for 7 days
2. Recombinant factor VIII 50 units/kg (IV) every 24 hours for 5 days

We decided on completing all the dental procedures on the same day based on the rigorous regimen the patient would need to go through to complete his dental treatment as most of his procedures required following the above protocol.

As far as the replacement of missing teeth, patient made an informed decision to have 3-unit bridge each to replace his missing teeth, as he did not want to have to go through the whole management process multiple times.

Hemophilia A (also Factor VIII deficiency, classic hemophilia) is a deficiency of the coagulation Factor VIII. This condition could be hereditary or acquired in origin and depending on severity, patients with this condition can present with life-threatening hemorrhage, including from intraoral sites.

Hereditary hemophilia A is an X-linked recessive disorder with disease typically manifesting in males, and females serving as carriers. This is the most common hereditary coagulation disorder, with 80% to 85% of hemophiliacs presenting with hemophilia A.[1] The severity of disease can be correlated with Factor VIII levels.

Acquired hemophilia A occurs as a result of immunoglobulin G autoantibodies/inhibitors formed against endogenous Factor VIII and has no sex predilection. This rare autoimmune condition typically occurs in elderly patients and could be associated with comorbid conditions such as rheumatoid arthritis, malignancies, and infections. In younger people, pregnancy is the highest risk factor.[2] Factor VIII levels do not always correlate with disease severity in acquired hemophilia A.

Most dentists are uncomfortable with treating patients with hemophilia, as minor trauma can result in life-threatening complications. However, in consult with a hematologist, some patients can be treated in an outpatient environment, whereas others will require inpatient hospital treatment. This decision is based on disease severity and the dental procedure to be performed. The hematologist would typically propose a management plan that is specific to the patient, which the dentist should be aware of.

Preventive oral care is pivotal in patients with hemophilia A to avoid the need for invasive dental procedures. Implants are also not an absolute contraindication in patients with hemophilia. However, risk–benefit has to be assessed to make informed decisions.[2]

Radiograph placement in the oral cavity should be done with caution so as not to cause minor injuries that can result in complications. An aspiration syringe has to be used with injecting local anesthesia. Caution also has to be used with inferior alveolar nerve blocks, and lingual infiltration is avoided due to the high vascularity in that area. Local hemostatic measures should be used after procedures, for example, suturing at extraction sites, even when bleeding is not immediately observed. It should be kept in mind that bleeding is delayed in patients with coagulation disorders. A 24-hour post-treatment follow-up is also recommended after all dental procedures, especially those involving tissue manipulation.[3]

CLINICS CARE POINTS

- Preventive dental care should be included in the managment plan of patients with hemophilia.
- Patients with hemophila can be treated in an outpatient dental clinic, especially for dental procedures not requiring tissue manipulation, however consulting with a hematologist is highly recommended.

REFERENCES

1. Mehta P, Reddivari AKR. In: Hemophilia. FL: StatPearls Publishing; Treasure Island; 2022.
2. Kruse-Jarres R, Kempton CL, Baudo F, et al. Acquired hemophilia A: updated review of evidence and treatment guidance. Am J Hematol 2017;92(7):695–705.
3. Abed H, Ainousa A. Dental management of patients with inherited bleeding disorders: a multidisciplinary approach. Gen Dent 2017;56–60.

Patient with von Willebrand Disease Presenting for Selective Scaling and Root Planning

Temitope T. Omolehinwa, BDS, DMD, DScD[a],*,
Adeyinka Dayo, BDS, DMD, MS[a], Enitan Adegite, MD, MPH[b]

KEYWORDS

- von Willebrand disease • von Willebrand factor
- Dental management of von Willebrand disease

KEY POINTS

- Patients with von Willebrand disease can besuccessfully treated in a dental setting.
- Treating patients with vWD requires consultation with a hematologist especially when invasive dental treatments are planned.
- von Willebrand disease is acquired or congenital.

MEDICAL SCENARIO

A 74-year-old White woman presents to the dental clinic following referral from an outside periodontist, with chief complaint of pain in her maxillary anterior area. She recently had multiple crowns placed on her maxillary arch and was experiencing pain especially between her upper left central and lateral incisors (teeth #9 and #10).

Medical history was positive for von Willebrand disease (vWD), type II diabetes, history of a transischemic attack with coronary stent placement, and depression. Her medications include glipizide, pravastatin, venlafaxine, and atenolol. She reports multiple hematomas and 80% deafness in her left ear. She reports multiple surgeries with postoperative bleeding complications that happened before her diagnosis of vWD.

On intraoral examination, there was grade 2 mobility on #10, with #9 and #10 positive to percussion. Also noted was erythema on lingual gingiva of #9. Intraoral

[a] Penn Dental Medicine, University of Pennsylvania, Philadelphia, PA, USA; [b] Drexel University, St Christopher's Children Hospital, Philadelphia, PA, USA
* Corresponding author. Oral Medicine Department, Room 212 Schattner Buiding, 240 South 40th Street, Philadelphia, PA 19104.
E-mail address: omote@upenn.edu

Dent Clin N Am 67 (2023) 469–472
https://doi.org/10.1016/j.cden.2023.02.023
0011-8532/23/© 2023 Elsevier Inc. All rights reserved.

radiograph showed significant vertical bone loss between #9 and #10, and a radio-opacity indicative of an overhang mesial of #10 on the root surface (**Fig. 1**).

DENTAL MANAGEMENT DECISION AND JUSTIFICATION

Dental management plan included deep scaling by open flap surgery with direct debridement or conventional deep scaling, to remove the overhang noted as radio-opacity on the radiograph. She also required periodontal probing, postponed for after hematology consultation.

Before the procedure, the patient's hematologist was consulted. This should be the first step in managing patients with bleeding disorders, especially hereditary disorders.

The treatment protocol for management of vWD is patient specific and depends on disease severity. The patient described previously has type 2 vWD. Her treatment protocol included intravenous desmopressin (DDAVP) the morning of dental procedure requiring tissue manipulation and then follow-up with her hematologist postprocedure to evaluate postprocedural bleeding and need for either more DDAVP or tranexamic acid tablet.

We were able to deep scale with a piezo ultrasonic scaler and remove the overhang, which was noted as excess cement. Patient followed up with her hematologist and needed another dose of desmopressin same day. Patient returned 2 weeks later; the pain had resolved, and so did the gingival erythema.

vWD is a platelet phase bleeding disorder, affecting platelet aggregation and adhesion. It is inherited or acquired in origin.[1] Acquired vWD is usually as a result of

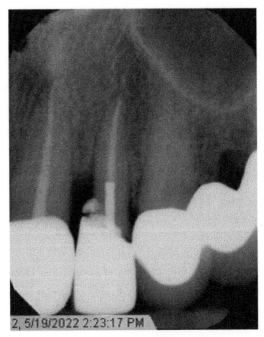

Fig. 1. Intraoral periapical radiograph showing multiple crowns on #9–11 and a pontic in place of #12. Teeth #9 and #10 are root canal treated with a post on #10. There is a radiopaque overhang material mesial of #10, which was causing pain.

lymphoproliferative diseases, cardiac disorders, myeloproliferative diseases, medications, autoimmune conditions, solid tumors, hypothyroidism, or specific medications,[2] resulting in impaired von Willebrand factor (vWF). The inherited vWD is the most common inherited bleeding disorder.

vWF is a glycoprotein that is found on the surfaces of platelets and factor VIII and vWD could result from decreased number or presence of nonfunctional vWF. vWD does not have any sex predilection. Type I vWD is the most common and with the least severity, affecting 70% to 80% of patients. When inherited, types 1 and 2 are autosomal-dominant diseases.

There are four different variants of type 2 vWD: 2A, 2B, 2N, and 2M. Type 3 vWD is the least common disease with the most severity, affecting factor FVIII and platelet activity.[3] It is also an autosomal-recessive disease, when inherited. Patients with types 2N and 3 could present with hemophilia-like symptoms.

Diagnosis of vWD is typically from a combination of clinical symptoms and/or laboratory tests including but not limited to vWF antigen, vWF ristocetin cofactor activity, factor VIII activity, complete blood counts,[4] and multimer assays.[2] Multimer assays determine the specific type 2 variant.

Treatment usually includes desmopressin and in severe cases von vWF/FVIII concentrate or recombinant vWF.[4] vWD types 1, 2A, and 2M are treated with desmopressin, whereas types 2N and 3 are unresponsive to desmopressin and require vWF/FVIII concentrate.[4,5]

Although management of patients with vWD could frighten dentists unfamiliar with this condition, these patients are effectively managed without complications when managed in consult with the hematologist. Some considerations include reinforcing preventive care to avoid the need for invasive procedures, use of an aspiration syringe when giving local anesthesia, and careful placement of radiograph in the oral cavity so as not to cause minor injuries that can result in complications. Caution also must be used with inferior alveolar nerve blocks, and lingual infiltration should be avoided because of the high vascularity in that area. Local hemostatic measures should be used after procedures (eg, considering use of periopak after scaling and root planning or scaling a few teeth to a quadrant at a time, to avoid multiple areas of bleeding). A 24-hour follow-up should also be encouraged for all patients with vWD. A patient-specific protocol recommended by the hematologist is followed for each patient.

CLINICS CARE POINTS

- Preventive oral care is highly encouraged in patients with vWD, to avoid bleeding complications associated with invasive dental treatment.
- It is advisable than any procedures requiring tissue manipulation should be done after consult with the hematologist.

REFERENCES

1. Sabih A, Babiker HM. Von Willebrand disease. In: StatPearls. Treasure Island (FL): StatPearls Publishing; 2022. Available at: https://www.ncbi.nlm.nih.gov/books/NBK459222/.
2. Franchini M, Mannucci PM. Acquired von Willebrand syndrome: focused for hematologists. Haematologica 2020;105(8):2032-7.

3. Swami A, von Willebrand Disease Kaur V. A concise review and update for the practicing physician. Clin Appl Thromb Hemost 2017;23(8):900–10.
4. Leebeek FW, Eikenboom JC. Von Willebrand disease. N Engl J Med 2016;375(21): 2067–80.
5. De Padua V, Romeo U, Santoro C, et al. Dental invasive procedures in von Willebrand disease outpatients treated with high purity FVIII/VWF complex concentrate (Fanhdi®): experience of a single center. Heliyon 2020;6(2):e03426.

Young Hemophilia Patient Presenting with Avulsed Maxillary Permanent Incisor

Jayakumar Jayaraman, BDS, MDS, FDSRCS, MS, PhD

KEYWORDS

- Hemophilia A • Bleeding • Factor VIII • Children • Avulsion • Dental treatment

KEY POINTS

- Hemophilia A is an x-linked recessive genetic condition characterized by Factor VIII deficiency.
- As children with hemophilia are more prone to bleeding from dental procedures, a hematologist must be consulted before dental procedures.
- Factor VIII replacement therapy levels must be checked, and any medications that might interfere with the coagulation process must be avoided.

MEDICAL SCENARIO

Young hemophilia patient presenting with avulsed maxillary permanent incisor.

A 7-year-old girl presented with a complaint of "My upper front tooth knocked out while I slipped and fell on the floor playing with my dog". She had her permanent maxillary central incisors, teeth #8 and #9 avulsed 45 minutes back. Bleeding was controlled by biting on a wet cloth. The avulsed teeth were immediately placed in a cup of milk. The caretaker did not report loss of consciousness. Tetanus immunization was up to date.

The patient had an established dental home, clinically caries-free with fair oral hygiene. The mother reports that the child was diagnosed with mild hemophilia A (>5% Factor VIII) immediately after birth. The child is regularly seen by a hematologist and the Factor VIII levels are within normal levels with adequate daily supplementation. There was no recent history of uncontrolled bleeding or trauma-related hospital visits. She reported no known drug or food allergy.

Medications included recombinant antihemophilic factor 20 IU/kg body weight IV three times a week.

Pediatric Dentistry, Children's Hospital of Richmond, Suite 200, Floor 6, 1000 East Broad Street, Richmond, VA 23219, USA
E-mail address: jayakumar83@hotmail.com

Dent Clin N Am 67 (2023) 473–476
https://doi.org/10.1016/j.cden.2023.02.021
0011-8532/23/© 2023 Elsevier Inc. All rights reserved.

On clinical exam, she was brachycephalic, of convex profile, and no facial asymmetry. No extraoral injuries were noted. The patient was conscious and responsive to pupillary response. All cranial nerves were intact.

Intraoral exam with mixed dentition. Overjet of 4 mm. Missing (avulsed) teeth # 8, 9, and the socket was covered with a clot, mild gingival laceration. No mobility or fracture was observed in the other maxillary or mandibular anterior teeth. An uncomplicated crown fracture involving enamel and dentin of teeth #8,9.

Three periapical radiographs were taken at different angles focused on avulsed teeth #8, 9. The socket corresponding to the teeth was intact with a normal alveolar bone pattern, and no crown or root fractures were observed in adjacent maxillary anterior teeth. A diagnosis of avulsion with uncomplicated fracture of teeth #8, 9 was rendered.

The patient had a Frankl Behavior Rating Scale 3 (Positive)—Acceptance of treatment, at times curious, willing to comply with the dentist.

DENTAL MANAGEMENT DECISION AND JUSTIFICATION

Based on previous history of trauma and current clotting potential observed in the socket, the teeth were immediately replanted and splinted. The patient was referred to hematology for follow-up. Medical consultation was not obtained at the time of replantation due to the time constraint of extra-oral time. A consult was sent to the hematologist for future dental treatments. The child has been diagnosed with mild hemophilia A (>5% Factor VIII level). The patient is taking recombinant antihemophilic Factor VIII three times a week. The factor levels and activated partial thromboplastin time (A-PTT) are within normal limits.

For anxiolysis, nitrous oxide and oxygen sedation were used at the ratio of 40:60. Benzocaine 20% was applied for topical anesthesia, and 2% Lidocaine (1:100,000 Epinephrine) was given as infiltration around the socket of the teeth # 8, 9 (4.4 mg/kg body weight). The socket was gently cleaned with a sterile saline solution. The teeth were taken from the milk, gently cleaned with sterile saline, and replanted in the socket. The position of the tooth in the socket was verified and occlusion was checked. Following this, teeth #7, 8, 9, 10 were splinted with 0.016″ stainless steel wire and packable composite resin restoration (**Fig. 1**). A periapical radiograph was taken to ensure adequate placement of the replanted teeth (**Fig. 2**). Post-operative instructions given included a soft diet, gentle cleaning with a soft brush, and anticipatory guidance on trauma prevention. Amoxicillin 30 mg/kg body weight was prescribed orally three times daily for 5 days. Acetaminophen (Tylenol) was prescribed for pain as needed. Hemostasis was confirmed before discharge. The patient was seen after

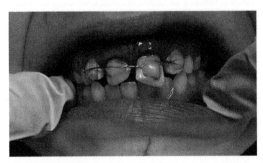

Fig. 1. Avulsed maxillary central incisors, teeth #8,9 replanted and splinted with 0.016″ stainless steel wire and resin composite.

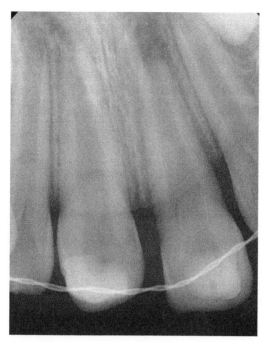

Fig. 2. Periapical radiograph shows adequate position of the permanent central incisors, teeth #8,9 with immature root following replantation.

2 weeks for splint removal that showed good healing of soft tissues and the teeth were stable (**Fig. 3**).

Hemophilia A is an x-linked recessive hereditary disorder that characterizes in three forms based on Factor VIII: severe (<1%), moderate (1%–5%), and mild (6%–50%).[1] The severity of bleeding depends on the amount of Factor VIII in plasma and the treatment modality following dental trauma must be planned based on the type of hemophilia A. Management of avulsion injury is time-dependent and it has been shown that periodontal ligament fibers tend to lose their vitality if the extra-oral time exceeds 60 minutes.[2] Hence, in this patient, it was decided to replant the teeth before consultation with a hematologist. The risk of leaving the teeth outside the socket and the time taken benefit of hematologist consultation or bleeding test must be balanced depending on the severity of hemophilia and current Factor VIII levels. A thorough medical

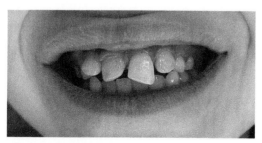

Fig. 3. Photograph taken at 2 weeks after splint removal showing good healing of soft tissue and stable maxillary central incisors.

history must be sought for patients who have had dental trauma, particularly pertaining to hemophilia. This includes history of bleeding control, loss of consciousness, and immunization. The level of consciousness is obtained by pupillary response and cranial nerve evaluation. To prevent the possibility of acquired tetanus, a booster is recommended if the last dose exceeds 5 years. For all avulsed teeth, antibiotics must be prescribed as a standard infection prevention protocol.[3] The choice of splinting material depends on the provider, ideally 0.25 mm (0.016″) stainless steel wire or a 40-pound composite fishing line cemented with packable resin composite material. The splinting must be removed at 2 weeks as a longer duration of splinting might result in ankylosis. In this patient, the prognosis of the treatment is considered guarded to fair as avulsed teeth #8, 9 had an immature root and the tooth replanted within a 1-hour time frame. Anticipatory guidance on trauma prevention was provided and it was recommended to use a mouthguard when engaging in contact sport.

REFERENCES

1. Yee R, Duggal MS, Wong VYY, et al. An Update on the Dental Management of Children with Haemophilia. Prim Dent J 2021;10(4):45–51.
2. Fouad AF, Abbott PV, Tsilingaridis G, et al. International Association of Dental Traumatology guidelines for the management of traumatic dental injuries: 2. Avulsion of permanent teeth. Dent Traumatol 2020;36(4):331–42.
3. Shastry SP, Kaul R, Baroudi K, et al. Hemophilia A: Dental considerations and management. J Int Soc Prev Community Dent 2014;4(Suppl 3):S147–52.

Mandibular Arteriovenous Malformation (Vascular Lesion) in a 16-Year-Old Patient

Adeyinka Dayo, BDS, DMD, MS*,
Temitope T. Omolehinwa, BDS, DMD, DScD

KEYWORDS

- Vascular neoplasm • Arteriovenous malformation • Bleeding • Embolization

KEY POINTS

- Vascular lesion/disease should be suspected when there is unexplained bleeding from the oral cavity.
- Importance of diagnostic imaging in patient management.
- Acknowledgement of expertise/limitation, and knowing when the need for referral arises.

MEDICAL SCENARIO

A 16-year-old girl presents to the dental clinic with persistent oozing of blood from the right posterior mandible and slight right side facial asymmetry. The patient claims to have had two other similar episodes from her right first mandibular molar tooth region, which were nonconsequential, and thought to be part of puberty. She denies history of trauma, pain, or dental infection. Family history was unremarkable and review of systems was noncontributory. Intraoral examination revealed an epulis on the buccal gingiva adjacent to the crown of the right first mandibular molar and active bleeding from the gingival margin of the second premolar and second molar in the same region. Panoramic radiograph obtained as part of the evaluation process revealed an irregular widening of the right inferior alveolar canal, extending from the mandibular foramen to mental foramen and widening of the periodontal ligament space of the involved teeth.

DENTAL MANAGEMENT DECISION AND JUSTIFICATION

The immediate management for this patient was controlling her presenting symptom (pulsatile bleeding) by use of local hemostatic measures. In this case, pressure with

Department of Oral Medicine, University of Pennsylvania School of Dental Medicine, 240 South 40th Street, Philadelphia, PA 19104, USA
* Corresponding author. Department of Oral Medicine, University of Pennsylvania School of Dental Medicine, 240 South 40th Street, Philadelphia, PA 19140.
E-mail address: dayoad@upenn.edu

Dent Clin N Am 67 (2023) 477–479
https://doi.org/10.1016/j.cden.2023.02.024
0011-8532/23/© 2023 Elsevier Inc. All rights reserved.

dental.theclinics.com

sterile gauze packs was applied, while paramedics were called in to take the patient to an emergency room because a bleeding disorder was suspected. The paramedics arrived in time and therefore other methods of local hemostasis were not used. Other local hemostatic measures that could be used include rinsing with tranexamic acid rinse; suturing; or application of absorbable hemostats, such as oxidized regenerated cellulose, sealants, and fibrin adhesives.

At the emergency room, more diagnostic imaging studies were ordered including multidetector computed tomography, MRI, and magnetic resonance angiography. Findings confirmed the presence of an arteriovenous malformations in jaw (j-AVM).

Intraosseous j-AVMs are rare congenital high-flow vascular abnormalities regarded as fatal hemorrhagic disease in the maxillofacial region.[1,2] AVM has an estimated prevalence of 1/100,000 person-years, and j-AVMs are rare.[2] Although rare, j-AVM may be life threatening if inadvertently unveiled by a tooth extraction or biopsy, and lead to profuse, exsanguinating hemorrhage.

Several theories have been postulated as to the cause of AVM, one of which is that it is caused by errors in embryogenesis,[3,4] causing progressive expansion of abnormal vessels lined by flat endothelium. These vessels are present at birth and grow proportionately with the child.

Diagnostic imaging is a valuable tool in diagnosing and localizing vascular lesions. AVM has characteristic radiographic features that if combined with the clinical signs and symptoms may aid diagnosis. Radiographically, the lesion may present as irregular periapical radiolucency centered on a tooth, multilocular radiolucency with a "soap-bubble" appearance in the mandibular body and ramus, mimicking cystic or tumoral jaw lesions, or irregular widening and enlargement of the mandibular canal with a serpiginous course. Multidetector computed tomography, MRI, magnetic resonance angiography and superselective arteriography are essential tools for localization of the arteriovenous shunt and treatment planning.[5]

Management of AVM is complex and requires a multidisciplinary approach. Treatment may span superselective angiographic embolization to surgical resection of the involved bone.[2,4,5] Relapse after treatment can occur and intraosseous injection of sclerosing agents may be used to reduce the number of arterial embolization.[5]

A patient with facial swelling and unexplained bleeding from the oral cavity should be suspected to have a bleeding disorder. The spontaneous, pulsatile bleeding and depressible, floating tooth observations are characteristic of hemangiomas or AVMs. No invasive dental treatment should be performed on this patient until the diagnosis of a vascular pathology is ruled out. Other intraoral features may include epulis, toothache, loose or floating tooth, and gingival swelling.

Another consideration is the importance of recognizing the clinical presentation of unexplained bleeding in the oral cavity. The dentist should not be in a rush to perform invasive dental treatment until the source of bleeding is identified.

CLINICS CARE POINTS

- Need for comprehensive history of presenting complain.
- Need for documentation of medical and surgical history.
- Importance of appropriate diagnostic imaging.

REFERENCES

1. Li X, Su L, Wang D, et al. Clinical and imaging features of intraosseous arteriovenous malformations in jaws: a 15-year experience of single centre. Sci Rep 2020; 10(1):12046.
2. Rosen RJ, Nassiri N, Drury JE. Interventional management of high-flow vascular malformations. Tech Vasc Interv Radiol 2013;16(1):22–38.
3. Higuera S, Gordley K, Metry DW, et al. Management of hemangiomas and pediatric vascular malformations. J Craniofac Surg 2006;17(4):783–9.
4. Noreau G, Landry P Moreau, Morais D. Arteriovenous malformation of the mandible: review of literature and case history. J Can Dent Assoc 2001;67(11): 646–51.
5. Spreafico R, Sordo L, Bellotto R, et al. Arterio-venous malformation of the mandible. Case report and review of literature. Acta Otorhinolaryngol Ital 2016; 36(4):333–6.

Patient Living with Human Immunodeficiency Virus and Depression with High HIV Viral Load Presenting for Evaluation of Root Caries

Temitope T. Omolehinwa, BDS, DMD, DScD[a],*,
Osamudiamen Idahosa, MD[b], Chizobam Idahosa, BDS, DDS, MS[c]

KEYWORDS

• HIV • HIV RNA/viral load • High viral load

KEY POINTS

- Patients with HIV with high HIV viral load only, do not need modifications in dental management.
- HIV is now a chronic medical conditions, with most patients having stable disease if they are compliant with their medications.
- Universal infection control protocols should be followed for all patients regardless of their HIV status.

MEDICAL SCENARIO

A 26-year-old man presents to the dental clinic with chief complaint of sensitivity to cold foods or drinks affecting his lower left posterior teeth of 2 weeks duration. His medical history is positive for HIV for which he is treated with combination antiretroviral therapy: elvitegravir, cobicistat, emtricitabine, and tenofovir alafenamide. He sees a psychologist for symptoms of depression. He had been compliant with his medications since his diagnosis 6 years ago. However, in the last month, because of work-related issues, he skipped several doses of his medication.

Intraoral examination revealed lower left first molar (tooth #19) buccal surface with root caries below the gingival margin.

[a] Department of Oral Medicine, Penn Dental Medicine University of Pennsylvania, Room 212 Schattner Building, 240 South 40th Street, Philadelphia, PA 19104, USA; [b] Department of Critical Care Medicine, St Luke's University Health Network, Bethlehem, PA 18015, USA; [c] Department of Oral Medicine, Penn Dental Medicine, Philadelphia, PA, USA
* Corresponding author.
E-mail address: omote@upenn.edu

Dent Clin N Am 67 (2023) 481–482
https://doi.org/10.1016/j.cden.2023.02.025
0011-8532/23/© 2023 Elsevier Inc. All rights reserved.

Table 1 Pertinent patient laboratory values		
Laboratory Study	**Patient Result**	**Normal Value**
Platelet count	170,000	150,000–400,000 cells/mL
Absolute neutrophil count	4350	1500–8000 cells/mL
CD4$^+$ count	320	500–1500 cells/mL
Viral load	130,000	Undetectable copies/mL

DENTAL MANAGEMENT DECISION AND JUSTIFICATION

A treatment plan for a resin restoration on #19 buccal was discussed with the patient. As is standard of practice for all patients with a known diagnosis of HIV, the following laboratory studies were requested: complete blood count with differentials, HIV viral load, and CD4$^+$ count. His laboratory study results are highlighted in **Table 1**. In regards to his slightly high viral load, there is no need for treatment modification in this patient, because a high viral load is not a direct indicator of how he will respond to dental treatment.[1]

Patients living with HIV should not be refused treatment only because of a high HIV viral load or a low CD4$^+$ cell count. Dentists should always remember that the determinants for dental management of patients living with HIV is based on absolute neutrophil and platelet counts (risk of infection and hemorrhage). Standard infection control protocols should always be used in dentistry regardless of HIV status of patients.

CLINICS CARE POINTS

- Depression is a common psychiatric finding in patients living with HIV.
- Depression, depending on severity, can lead to poor oral outcomes due to lack of motivation for self-care.

FUNDING

Grant #: R01DE029648 (NIH/NIDCR).

REFERENCES

1. Robbins MR. Recent recommendations for management of human immunodeficiency virus-positive patients. Dent Clin North Am 2017;61(2):365–87.

Dental Extraction in a Patient Living with Human Immunodeficiency Virus with Neutropenia and Thrombocytopenia

Temitope T. Omolehinwa, BDS, DMD, DScD[a],*,
Osamudiamen Idahosa, MD, FCCP[b],
Chizobam Idahosa, BDS, DDS, MS[a]

KEYWORDS

- HIV • Absolute neutrophil count (ANC) • Low platelets • Thrombocytopenia

KEY POINTS

- HIV patients with low platelet counts may require platelet transfusion before invasive dental treatment
- HIV patients with absolute neutrophil count less than 500 cells/mm³ require antibiotic coverage before dental treatment
- Modifications to dental treatment should not be based solely on HIV Ribonucleic acid (RNA) (viral load) and CD4+ cell count

MEDICAL SCENARIO

A 34-year-old male presents to the dental clinic following a referral from an oral medicine specialist for evaluation of throbbing tooth pain. Pain was noted to be in his upper right anterior area and had been present for a week. It was aggravated by hot and cold foods and severe enough to wake him up from sleep.

His medical history was positive for HIV/Acquired Immune Deficiency Syndrome (AIDS) and his medications included a combined antiretroviral therapy regimen (bictegravir/emtricitabine/tenofovir) and sulfamethoxazole/trimethoprim. He had an allergy to penicillin. Clinical examination revealed retained root of #6 (**Fig. 1**), which was

[a] Department of Oral Medicine, Penn Dental Medicine, University of Pennsylvania, 240 South 40th Street, Philadelphia, PA 19104, USA; [b] Department of Critical Care Medicine, St Luke's University Health Network, Bethlehem, PA, USA
* Corresponding author.
E-mail address: omote@upenn.edu

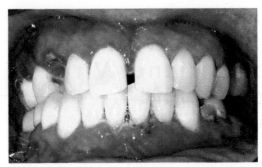

Fig. 1. Clinical picture of #6 with fractured crown up to gingival margin and tooth discoloration on #21 and crown fracture. Generalized gingival inflammation and ulceration of the interdental papillae between mandibular anterior teeth in a patient living with HIV.

tender to percussion; #21 was also grossly carious, fractured, and discolored from a necrotic pulp; #21 was non-responsive to cold pulp testing.

Further soft tissue examination showed generalized gingival inflammation and ulceration between the interdental papillae of #23 and #24. However, periodontal probing depths were normal and no attachment loss was noted. The patient reported that the referring oral medicine specialist prescribed chlorhexidine oral rinse and a systemic antibiotic.

DENTAL MANAGEMENT DECISION AND JUSTIFICATION

His treatment plan included gross debridement and extractions of non-restorable teeth #6 and #21. Before initiating dental treatment, we requested his current laboratory results. They were easily accessible on his phone.

On review of results, the patient was noted to have laboratory data consistent with AIDS. The criteria for AIDS diagnosis are laboratory evidence of HIV-1 or HIV-2 plus CD4+ count less than 200 cells/mm^3 or the presence of an AIDS-defining illness.[1] He also had thrombocytopenia and neutropenia (**Table 1**), with an increased risk of bleeding and infection during dental treatment.

Modifications to his dental treatment were based on his medical complexity, not his HIV status, as medically stable asymptomatic HIV patients do not require modifications before dental treatment.

Pertinent to the patient's laboratory finding of significant thrombocytopenia, we consulted with his physician and requested additional coagulation studies, including prothrombin time (PT)/international normalized ratio (INR) to evaluate additional bleeding risks before extractions. Results on PT/INR were normal, and it was agreed that teeth would be extracted one tooth at a time with local hemostatic measures, including suture use at the extraction site.[2] His management plan included

1. Azithromycin 600 mg stat, to be taken an hour before extraction (patient presented with ANC of 480 cells/mm3 and penicillin allergy)
2. Twenty-four hours post-procedure observation to evaluate for post-extraction bleeding

Antibiotic coverage is recommended for severely neutropenic patients with ANC of less than 500 cells/mL.[3] The decision for prophylactic antibiotics coverage should not be solely based on the CD4 count or viral load.[3] Post-procedural antibiotic coverage

Table 1
Patient's laboratory value, normal value, and implications for dental treatment

Laboratory Study	Patient Value	Normal Range	Implications for Dental Treatment
ANC	480	1500–8000 cells/mm^3	• Essential for assessing risk for bacterial infection and risk from invasive procedures • Neutrophils function as the first line of defense against bacterial infection. • Antibiotic prophylaxis recommended at ANC <500
Platelet count	40,000	150,000–400,000 cells/mm^3	• HIV can suppress the bone marrow resulting in hematologic abnormalities, including thrombocytopenia. Thrombocytopenia can also result as a side effect of antiretroviral therapy (ART) • Platelet replacement therapy may be needed with platelet counts <50,000 before invasive procedure
CD4+ cells	98	500–1500 cells/mL	• Marker of immune system competence and level of immunosuppression • Predictor of HIV-associated opportunistic infections • Dental patients should NOT be declined care or put on antibiotics solely based on CD4+
HIV viral load	3 million	Undetectable	• Marker of viral replication and level of infectivity • Predictor of disease progression due to CD4+ cell death • Guides selection of ART • Dental patients should NOT be declined care solely based on the HIV viral load

Patient's laboratory values with normal ranges, and implications for dental management.

was not given in this case because the patient was already on trimethoprim/sulfamethoxazole. If the patient had not been on antibiotics, post-procedural antibiotics would have been prescribed.

In addition, if the patient had a platelet count of less than 30,000 cells/mm^3, platelet transfusion would have been highly recommended. This is because of the high risk of spontaneous bleeding at platelet levels less than 30,000 cells/mm^3.

Dental treatment should never be withheld because of high viral load as patient–health care provider transmission risks are low if universal infection control standards are adhered to. Dentists are expected to adhere strictly to standard/universal precautions for infection control with every patient encounter, regardless of HIV status.

In the antiretroviral therapy (ART) era, HIV is now grouped in the category of chronic illnesses as most patients experience viral suppression evidenced by normal/near normal laboratory findings. Objective assessment of individual patients, and employing necessary precautions to avoid dental complications, are paramount in the management of patients living with HIV with thrombocytopenia and neutropenia. Before initiating any invasive dental treatment in a patient living with HIV, it is important to evaluate pertinent laboratory studies. Medical consult with the treating infectious disease specialist may be warranted, especially in patients with AIDS.

CLINICS CARE POINTS

- Routine complete blood count (CBC) should be reviewed at least annually, in patients living with HIV/AIDS receiving dental treatment.
- Patients with HIV should never be denied dental care based on a high HIV RNA/Viral load, or low CD4+ counts less than 200 cells/mL.

FUNDING

Grant number: R01DE029648 NIH/NIDCR.

REFERENCES

1. Centers for Disease Control and Prevention. AIDS and opportunistic infections. Available at: https://www.cdc.gov/hiv/basics/livingwithhiv/opportunisticinfections.html. Accessed on 09/12/2022.
2. Fillmore WJ, Leavitt BD, Arce K. Dental extraction in the thrombocytopenic patient is safe and complications are easily managed. JOMS 2013;71(10):1647–52.
3. Robbins MR. Recent recommendations for management of human immunodeficiency virus-positive patients. Dent Clin North Am 2017;61(2):365–87.

A 50-Year-Old Woman Living with Human Immunodeficiency Virus and Comorbid Conditions, Presenting for Scaling and Root Planing

Temitope T. Omolehinwa, BDS, DMD, DScD[a],*,
Osamudiamen Idahosa, MD, FCCP[b],
Chizobam Idahosa, BDS, DDS, MS[c]

KEYWORDS

- HIV • HIV-associated noninfectious comorbid conditions
- HIV-associated infectious comorbid conditions

KEY POINTS

- Modifications to dental treatment should not be based solely on HIV RNA (viral load) and CD4[+] cell count.
- Noninfectious comorbid conditions especially diabetes, cardiovascular disease, and hyperlipidemia are common findings in patients with HIV.
- Patients living with HIV are at high risk of infectious comorbid conditions, such as hepatitis C.
- Dentists can play a role in ensuring patients' comorbid medical conditions are well managed.

MEDICAL SCENARIO

A 50-year-old woman presents to the dental clinic with chief complaint of bleeding gums, especially with tooth brushing. She also reports some areas of swelling involving her gingivae and mobile teeth.

She came to the clinic with a summary sheet of her medical conditions, which included HIV, chronic hepatitis C with liver cirrhosis, poorly controlled diabetes,

[a] Department of Oral Medicine, Penn Dental Medicine University of Pennsylvania, Room 212 Schattner Building, 240 South 40th Street, Philadelphia, PA 19104, USA; [b] Department of Critical Care Medicine, St Luke's University Health Network, Bethlehem, PA 18015, USA; [c] Department of Oral Medicine, Penn Dental Medicine, University of Pennsylvania, Philadelphia, PA, USA
* Corresponding author.
E-mail address: omote@upenn.edu

Dent Clin N Am 67 (2023) 487–490
https://doi.org/10.1016/j.cden.2023.02.026
0011-8532/23/© 2023 Elsevier Inc. All rights reserved.

hyperlipidemia, and hypertension. Medications included dolutegravir, rilpivirine, atorvastatin, insulin glargine, insulin aspart, spironolactone, and nadolol.

Intraoral examination revealed multiple areas of deep pockets between 6 and 9 mm, clinical attachment loss in select posterior teeth, grade 1 to 2 mobility of some teeth, and a couple of teeth with periodontal abscesses.

DENTAL MANAGEMENT DECISION AND JUSTIFICATION

Treatment plan included scaling and root planing in all four quadrants with open debridement in specific areas.

Based on the number of comorbidities the patient presented with, her medical encounter notes and recent laboratory studies including complete blood count, complete metabolic panel, glycated hemoglobin, liver function tests, prothrombin time/international normalized ratio, and lipid panels were requested. The results of the laboratory studies are highlighted in **Table 1**. The encounter notes from her infectious disease specialist and primary care physician revealed most of her chronic illnesses were stable except for liver cirrhosis and uncontrolled diabetes.

Our medical management plan included the following.

- High blood pressure: Blood pressure measurements were recommended before dental procedures. Her blood pressure remained well controlled.
- Diabetes mellitus: Checking her blood glucose helps prevent hypoglycemia arising from use of rapid-acting (insulin aspart) and long-acting (insulin glargine) insulin during dental treatment. Other questions to ask are:
  - Did she eat before taking her insulin on the day of her procedure?
  - What is her normal blood glucose range?
  - What was the fasting blood sugar on the morning of her procedure?
  - What symptoms does she experience during a hypoglycemic episode?

We recommended she make us aware of any symptoms immediately.

Because of the patient's glycated hemoglobin of 11%, we recommended antibiotic coverage before and after scaling and root planning, because patients with poorly controlled diabetes have a high infection risk and poor wound healing.[1]

- Chronic hepatitis C and liver cirrhosis: Liver function tests, prothrombin time/international normalized ratio, and complete blood count should be periodically monitored for this patient. Cirrhosis staging (eg, Child-Pugh) assists in assessing risk for hemorrhagic complications, because patients with liver cirrhosis have a high risk of profound bleeding during procedures requiring tissue manipulation. Atraumatic technique and local hemostatic measures should be used to prevent bleeding complications. This can include scaling only one quadrant, instead of the full mouth at the first treatment visit, to reduce the risk of bleeding complications. Use of local hemostatic measures, and periodontal pack, may be needed if hemorrhage occurs. Because of hepatic metabolism, caution with local anesthesia dosing is recommended because of potential for toxicity.
- Hyperlipidemia: High-density lipoprotein and low-density lipoprotein should be monitored. The patient was well controlled on atorvastatin.
- HIV: There are no modifications purely based on the HIV diagnosis in this patient. It should be noted that the reason for providing antibiotic coverage to this patient is unrelated to her HIV status, but because of her uncontrolled diabetes.

Age-related HIV-associated noninfectious comorbid conditions are commonly seen among patients with HIV, with an earlier age of onset compared with age-matched

Table 1
Pertinent patient laboratory results for 50-year-old woman living with HIV who has other comorbid conditions

Blood Panel	Specific Test	Patient Value	Normal Range
Hepatitis C	Hep C DNA	870,000	Undetectable
Liver function tests	Aspartate aminotransferase	240	8–33 U/L
	Alanine aminotransferase	350	7–55 U/L
	Bilirubin	6	0.1–1.2 mg/dL
	Albumin	1.2	3.5–5.5 g/dL
Complete blood count with differentials	Platelets	80,000	150,000–450,000 cells/mm^3
	Absolute neutrophil count	1000	1500–8000 cells/mm^3
Bleeding tests	Prothrombin time	45	11.0–13.5 s
	International normalized ratio	3.1	<1.1
Immune panel	CD4$^+$	388	500–1500 cells/mm^3
	Viral load	<20	Undetectable
Complete metabolic panel	Glucose	280	70–100 mg/dL
	Glycated hemoglobin	11	<5.7%

HIV-naive patients.[2,3] The most prevalent conditions are metabolic diseases, such as hypertension, diabetes, and hyperlipidemia. Hepatitis C–HIV coinfection is reported in 21% of patients living with HIV.[4] Dentists can participate in routine evaluation of laboratory results and point patients toward timely evaluation by their physicians, because there have been cases where patients had abnormal laboratory results and had no knowledge of any problems because they had not scheduled follow-up visits to evaluate their results.

CLINICS CARE POINTS

- Patients with poorly controlled diabetes and periodontitis, should have both their disease treated simultaneously as poorly controlled diabetes is directly correlated with poor periodontal outcomes and vise versa.
- Hepatotoxic medications such asacetaminophen should be avoided in patients with liver cirrhosis.
- Patients with liver cirrhosis should be assessed for their bleeding risks prior to dental treatment requiring tissue manipulation.

FUNDING

Grant #: R01DE029648 (NIH/NIDCR).

REFERENCES

1. Miller A, Ouanounou A. Diagnosis, management, and dental considerations for the diabetic patient. JCan Dent Assoc 2020;86:k8.
2. Althoff K, Smit M, Reiss P, et al. HIV and ageing: improving quantity and quality of life. Curr Opin HIV AIDS 2016;11(5):527–36.
3. Marcus J, Leyden W, Alexeeff S, et al. Comparison of overall and comorbidity-free life expectancy between insured adults with and without HIV infection, 2000-2016. JAMA Netw Open 2020;3(6):e207954.
4. Centers for Disease Control (CDC). People co-infected with HIV and viral hepatitis. Available at: https://www.cdc.gov/hepatitis/populations/hiv. Assessed October 1, 2022.

Patient Living with Human Immunodeficiency Virus with a History of Chronic Obstructive Pulmonary Disease and Experiencing Oxygen Desaturation During Dental Treatment

Temitope T. Omolehinwa, BDS, DMD, DScD[a],*,
Osamudiamen Idahosa, MD, FCCP[b],
Chizobam Idahosa, BDS, DDS, MS[c]

KEYWORDS

- HIV • COPD • Chronic obstructive pulmonary disease

KEY POINTS

- Patients with a long smoking history have increased risk for chronic obstructive pulmonary disease (COPD).
- Nitrous oxide should be avoided in patients with COPD.
- Supplemental oxygen should be available and checked regularly for oxygen levels in dental settings, so they are available for use in emergencies.
- Patients with controlled HIV should be treated like any other controlled chronic illness.

MEDICAL SCENARIO

A 60-year-old Spanish-speaking man presented to the dental clinic for routine dental care with a chief complaint of "I have bad teeth and would like to fix them."

His medical history is positive for HIV for which he is being treated with Abacavir, and chronic obstructive pulmonary disease (COPD) for which he is being treated

[a] Department of Oral Medicine, Penn Dental Medicine University of Pennsylvania, Room 212 Schattner Building, 240 South 40th Street, Philadelphia, PA 19104, USA; [b] Department of Critical Care Medicine, St Luke's University Health Network, Bethlehem, PA 18015, USA; [c] Department of Oral Medicine, Penn Dental Medicine, University of Pennsylvania
* Corresponding author.
E-mail address: omote@upenn.edu

Dent Clin N Am 67 (2023) 491–493
https://doi.org/10.1016/j.cden.2023.02.027
0011-8532/23/© 2023 Elsevier Inc. All rights reserved.

dental.theclinics.com

with tiotropium (Spiriva), salmeterol, and albuterol/ipratropium (Combivent) as needed. He has no known allergies. His social history is positive for 30 pack-year cigarette smoking, and 5 to 6 bottles of beer a week. His review of systems is positive for intermittent shortness of breath.

He had a blood pressure of 124/88 mm Hg, pulse rate of 72 beats per minute, and oxygen saturation of 84% on room air. Repeated measures of his oxygen saturation were between 84% and 88%. The patient uses nocturnal 2 L supplemental oxygen. During history-taking, the patient began to experience a coughing bout and had symptoms of shortness of breath.

DENTAL MANAGEMENT DECISION AND JUSTIFICATION

At the patient's initial visit, because of the presenting oxygen saturation and symptoms, the authors placed him on 4 L/min of oxygen, delivered via a nasal cannula, and only discharged the patient to his wife when the oxygen saturation had bumped up to 95%.

A consult was then sent out to patient's pulmonologist as well as his primary care physician to obtain his recent pulmonology encounter notes and recent laboratory study results, respectively.

Review of his pulmonology encounter, which included results of his lung function and spirometry tests, showed severe disease. His FEV_1 (a measure of how much air a person can forcefully exhale in 1 second) was 32%. The patient's laboratory study results, including his complete blood count with differentials (especially absolute neutrophil and platelet counts), $CD4^+$ cell count, and HIV viral load, were all within normal limits. Although his HIV was well controlled, his COPD was not.

The authors' dental management plan included monitoring the patient's oxygen saturation throughout his dental visit using a pulse oximeter and giving supplemental oxygen when oxygen saturation fell below 90%. The authors also recommended that the patient bring his rescue albuterol/ipratropium inhaler each time he comes in for his appointment, for use when he has a coughing attack. Tobacco cessation education was also included on the management plan, and printed materials on tobacco cessation were handed to patient.

At the patient's subsequent visits, his oxygen levels with room air ranged from 82% to 93%. The patient was given 4 L/min supplemental oxygen by nasal cannula each time his oxygen levels on room air fell below 90%. The authors then continued with his dental care, which was completed uneventfully.

COPD, according to the American Lung Association, is a chronic lung condition that includes a combination of emphysema and chronic lung inflammation (chronic bronchitis).[1] Patients with COPD often have worsening respiratory symptoms, including shortness of breath and fatigue from airflow obstruction.[2]

Smoking is one of the most commonly known causes of COPD and is a preventable cause of this disease.

Tobacco smoking cessation education[3] is therefore an important tool to include in the dental care of patients with COPD, as oral care and oral disease prevention are discussed with patients.

Another factor to consider in the dental care of patients with COPD is that nitrous oxide cannot be used in this population, as it can cause respiration depression.[4]

Patients with severe COPD can be successful treated in an outpatient dental setting, and dentists are encouraged to ensure oxygen is readily available at the dental clinics in case of a respiratory emergency or other emergencies requiring supplemental oxygen administration.

CLINICS CARE POINTS

- Oral healthcare providers are encouraged to check oxygen saturation (O_2 sat.) in patients with COPD before initiating, and periodically during dental treatment.

- A patient with COPD presenting with O_2 sat. less than 90% in a dental setting, should first be asked to take deep breaths in, to see if this increases the O_2 levels.

- If taking deep breaths does not increase O_2 level, patient should be placed on 4-6L/min of O_2 to raise O_2 sat. to at least 90%.

FUNDING

Grant number: #R01DE029648 (NIDCR/NIH).

REFERENCES

1. American Lung Association. Available at: https://www.lung.org/lung-health-diseases/lung-disease-lookup/copd. Assessed on: 10/2/2022.
2. Labaki WW, Rosenberg SR. Chronic obstructive pulmonary disease. Ann Intern Med 2020;173(3):ITC17–32.
3. Rabe KF, Watz H. Chronic obstructive pulmonary disease. Lancet 2017; 389(10082):1931–40.
4. Rahman SS, Faruque M, Khan MHA, et al. Dental management of COPD patient. Bang Med J (Khulna) 2011;44:21–4.

Patient Living with Human Immunodeficiency Virus with Gingival Pain and Oral Soreness (Red and White Lesions)

Temitope T. Omolehinwa, BDS, DMD, DScD[a],*,
Osamudiamen Idahosa, MD, FCCP[b],
Chizobam Idahosa, BDS, DDS, MS[c]

KEYWORDS

- Candidiasis • HIV • Oral lesions in HIV • Necrotizing ulcerative gingivitis

KEY POINTS

- Patients with HIV with pseudomembranous or other forms of candidiasis are more likely to have AIDS.
- Recent laboratory findings of patients with HIV should be assessed to confirm their medical status.
- Patients with AIDS can present with necrotizing ulcerative gingivitis.
- Candidiasis in patients with HIV should be treated with systemic antifungals.
- Patients with necrotizing ulcerative gingivitis should be treated with topical and systemic antibiotics.

MEDICAL SCENARIO

A 34-year-old male presented to the oral medicine clinic for evaluation of throbbing gingival pain and oral soreness. He reported a 1-week history of constant pain involving the gingivae of multiple teeth, a fractured tooth, bleeding while brushing his teeth, foul breath, and generalized oral soreness. His past medical history is significant for HIV/AIDS disease, diagnosed 10 years before presentation.

Intraoral examination revealed diffuse, yellow, wipeable cottage-cheese–appearing plaques on erythematous palatal and buccal mucosa consistent with oral candidiasis (**Fig. 1**). There was generalized inflammation of the gingivae with bleeding on tissue manipulation, ulceration of the interdental papillae between mandibular anterior teeth,

[a] Department of Oral Medicine, Penn Dental Medicine, University of Pennsylvania, Room 212 Schattner Building, 240 South 40th Street, Philadelphia, PA 19104, USA; [b] Department of Critical Care Medicine, St Luke's University Health Network, Bethlehem, PA 18015, USA; [c] Department of Oral Medicine, Penn Dental Medicine, University of Pennsylvania
* Corresponding author.
E-mail address: omote@upenn.edu

Dent Clin N Am 67 (2023) 495–498
https://doi.org/10.1016/j.cden.2023.02.028
0011-8532/23/© 2023 Elsevier Inc. All rights reserved.

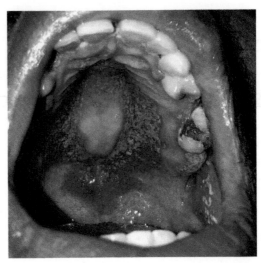

Fig. 1. Yellow, wipeable cottage-cheese–appearing plaques on erythematous palatal and buccal mucosa consistent with oral candidiasis, present in a patient living with HIV.

and class I mobility of mandibular anterior teeth with normal periodontal pocket depth and no clinical attachment loss, consistent with a diagnosis of necrotizing ulcerative gingivitis (NUG)[1] (**Fig. 2**).

DENTAL MANAGEMENT DECISION AND JUSTIFICATION

Oral candidiasis and NUG are oral manifestations of uncontrolled HIV.[2–4] The dentist should be concerned that the patient may have the most severe stage of HIV, AIDS. To assess the status of his HIV, the dentist should take a detailed history, including the following questions:

- How often and when last did you see your infectious disease specialist?
- Do you take your medications as prescribed?
- Have you received an AIDS diagnosis?
- How recently were your laboratory tests (blood work) updated? Do you have a printed copy or remote access from your phone?
- Have you been recently hospitalized for HIV-related complications?

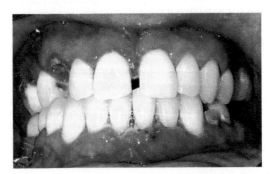

Fig. 2. Generalized gingival inflammation and ulceration of the interdental papillae between mandibular anterior teeth, in a patient living with HIV.

Table 1
Patients laboratory value

Laboratory Study	Patient Value	Normal Range
ANC, cells/mm^3	480	1500–8000
Platelet count, cells/mm^3	40,000	150,000–400,000
CD4$^+$ cells, cells/mL	98	500–1500 cells/mL
HIV viral load, copies/mL	3,000,000	Undetectable

Laboratory study findings (includes normal values) in a 34-year-old patient living with HIV.

The patient reported he had not been consistent with his medication in the past year, as he had been distracted with some emotional challenges. His recent laboratory studies from a couple of weeks before presentation were available on his phone, as seen in **Table 1**. It was obvious from the laboratory data that he had uncontrolled disease and needed to be more adherent to his HIV medication and be under close monitoring by his infectious disease doctor. This was discussed with the patient.

For his palatal lesions, the patient was treated with Fluconazole 100 mg tablets, taking 2 immediately and then 1 daily for 14 days. A systemic antifungal agent was prescribed owing to his immunocompromised state.[5] Immune-competent patients with mild oral candidiasis will benefit from Clotrimazole troches 10 mg, dissolving one slowly in the mouth 5 times a day.

In addition, the patient was prescribed Chlorhexidine gluconate 0.12%, an antimicrobial rinse and systemic antibiotics, 875 mg/125 mg Amoxicillin Clavulanate for his NUG. An alternative systemic antibiotic that can be used is Metronidazole with Penicillin VK.

The patient was then referred to the general dentist to take care of his dental needs noted during oral clinical examination. At the end of the visit, the authors also emphasized the need for follow-up with his infectious disease specialist.

CLINICS CARE POINTS

- Oral healthcare providers should identify oral manifestations of HIV/AIDS such as candidiasis, acute necrotizing ulcerative gingivitis, oral warts, etc; and refer patients appropriately for treatment
- The platelet and absolute neutrophil counts (components of the complete blood count), should be evaluated prior to dental treatment.

FUNDING

Grant #: R01DE029648 (NIDCR/NIH).

REFERENCES

1. Malek R, Gharibi A, Khlil N, et al. Necrotizing Ulcerative Gingivitis. Contemp Clin Dent 2017;8(3):496–500.
2. Mosca NG, Rose Hathorn A. HIV-positive patients: dental management considerations. Dent Clin North Am 2006;50(4):635–57.

3. Shekatkar M, Kheur S, Gupta AA, et al. Oral candidiasis in human immunodeficiency virus-infected patients under highly active antiretroviral therapy. Dis Mon 2021;67(9):101169.
4. Aškinytė D, Matulionytė R, Rimkevičius A. Oral manifestations of HIV disease: A review. Stomatologija 2015;17(1):21–8. PMID: 26183854.
5. Rajadurai SG, Maharajan MK, Veettil SK, et al. Comparative Efficacy of Antifungal Agents Used in the Treatment of Oropharyngeal Candidiasis among HIV-Infected Adults: A Systematic Review and Network Meta-Analysis. J Fungi (Basel) 2021; 7(8):637.

A Patient with Severe Anxiety and Episodes of Fainting in Need of Dental Restoration

Nikhil Mistry, DMD, MD[a], Kenneth Kufta, DMD, MD[a],
Mel Mupparapu, DMD, MDS[b],*, Neeraj Panchal, DMD, MD, MA[c]

KEYWORDS

- Syncope • Vasovagal episodes • Trendelenburg position • Facial pallor
- Ammonia inhalant

KEY POINTS

- Vasovagal or reflex syncope is often referred to as fainting.
- If a syncopal episode is suspected, the patient should be placed in a supine position with their legs elevated 10° (Trendelenburg position) above the head to increase cerebral perfusion.
- The patient's blood sugar should be assessed and treated as described below regarding hypoglycemic emergencies.

MEDICAL SCENARIO

A 24-year-old woman arrived alone to the dental clinic for continuation of her treatment plan following a prophylaxis (scaling and root planing of teeth) at her previous visit. The patient has several restorations remaining in all 4 quadrants of her mouth that need to be completed. She never had any prior restorations before and only had a cleaning performed by her hygienist over the years. The patient is planning on having tooth no. 18 restored with an occlusal resin restoration. Her medical history is significant for severe dental anxiety and previous syncopal episodes outside of the dental setting. The patient reports that her last syncopal episode was 5 months ago when she was at her primary care physician's office for the flu shot. The patient rates her dental anxiety a 10/10 and reports that her dental phobia is the reason she does not regularly visit the dental clinic. The patient denies any known drug

[a] Hospital of the University of Pennsylvania, Philadelphia, PA, USA; [b] Penn Dental Medicine, Philadelphia, PA, USA; [c] Penn Dental Medicine, Penn Presbyterian Medical Center, Philadelphia VA Hospitals, Philadelphia, PA, USA
* Corresponding author.
E-mail address: mmd@upenn.edu

Dent Clin N Am 67 (2023) 499–501
https://doi.org/10.1016/j.cden.2023.02.029
0011-8532/23/© 2023 Elsevier Inc. All rights reserved.

allergies. Within 5 minutes of seating the patient and updating her medical history, the dentist performs an examination. The patient quickly becomes tachycardic while endorsing lightheadedness and exhibits diaphoresis and facial pallor. The patient suddenly loses postural tone and consciousness while remaining reclined in the dental chair.

DENTAL MANAGEMENT

Given this presentation, the dentist should be concerned that the patient is experiencing a vasovagal syncopal episode. Vasovagal syncope accounts for over two-thirds of all medical emergencies in the dental office.[1,2] Syncope is characterized by a sudden loss of consciousness and loss of postural tone with rapid recovery (<2 minutes).[2,3] There are 3 main causes of syncope: vasovagal or reflex syncope, cardiac syncope, and syncope with neurologic causes. Vasovagal or reflex syncope, often referred to as fainting, is the most common form of syncope, and the type most often encountered in the dental setting. The occurrence of syncope is often elicited by many precipitants, including prolonged upright sitting, emotional and physical stressors, pain, dehydration, and use of vasodilators or diuretics.[2,3] Vasovagal syncope is often preceded by prodromal signs and symptoms, which can include facial pallor, diaphoresis, faintness, dizziness, lightheadedness, nausea or vomiting, warmth, tachycardia or bradycardia, and hypotension.[1-3] These early signs and symptoms are then typically followed by a loss of consciousness and postural tone resulting in collapse.[1,3] After the dentist recognizes a syncopal episode, it is crucial to promptly evaluate the patient in an organized fashion. Assessment of the patients' airway, breathing, and circulation (ABC's) per basic life support (BLS) protocol remains at the forefront of management of all medical emergencies. Immediate evaluation of ABC's should be completed to ensure the patient's airway is patent and without obstruction, their breathing is appropriate with adequate rise and fall of the chest, and their circulation is intact by palpation of the carotid or radial artery pulse.[4] If a syncopal episode is suspected, the patient should be placed in a supine position with their legs elevated 10° (Trendelenburg position) above the head to increase cerebral perfusion.[5] Supplemental oxygen (15 L/min) should be administered prophylactically via a nasal cannula,[2,6] and an aromatic ammonia inhalant can be held 4 to 6 inches under the patient's nose.[7]

Consciousness is typically regained in less than 2 minutes from the onset of symptoms. The patient's blood sugar should be assessed and treated as described below regarding hypoglycemic emergencies.[1] Continued patient monitoring before discharge is essential. If available, the patient should be escorted home by a responsible adult.[7] A postsyncopal phase can last hours and even several days in rare cases and thus continued monitoring is essential until the patient returns to their baseline. Symptoms of a postsyncopal phase could include nausea, dizziness, and an overall feeling of confusion or disorientation.[8] If consciousness is not regained within 2 minutes, other causes of loss of consciousness must be considered, including panic attack, seizure, cardiac pathologic conditions, metabolic derangements, or hypoglycemia.[9,10] Reassessment of the patient's ABC's and responsiveness should be regularly performed in the absence of consciousness. If any element of the patient's airway, breathing, or cardiovascular system is no longer intact, the provider should commence emergency BLS protocols and notify emergency medical services immediately.[11] The reported mortality in patients with a cardiac cause of syncope is 18% to 33%, and 0% to 12% in noncardiac causes.[11] Rapid recognition and response are crucial in preventing progression of more serious causes of syncope and in optimizing patient outcomes.

CLINICS CARE POINTS

- A syncopal attack is identified when the patient exhibits extreme anxiety in the dental chair followed by lighheadedness, diaphoresis and facial pallor leading to postural tone and consciousness.

- Assessment of airway, breathing and circulation is the first important step before placing the patient in a Trendelenburg position.

- Supplemental oxygen at a rate of 15 L/min should be administered via nasal canula along with an aromatic ammonia inhalant if available.

- Patient's blood sugar should also be assessed before dismissing with a responsible adult.

DISCLOSURE

The authors have nothing to disclose.

REFERENCES

1. Jevon P. Updated posters to help manage medical emergencies in the dental practice. Br Dent J 2015;219(5):227–9.
2. Hutse I, Coppens M, Herbelet S, et al. Syncope in dental practices: a systematic review on aetiology and management. J Evid Base Dent Pract 2021;21(3):101581.
3. da Silva RM. Syncope: epidemiology, etiology, and prognosis. Front Physiol 2014;5:471.
4. Palmer-Bouva C., Van R., de Vries R., et al., Fainting in the dental chair, *Oral Surg Oral Med Oral Pathol Oral Radiol Endod*, 86 (5), 1998, 508–510.
5. Malamed SF. Emergency medicine: beyond the basics. J Am Dent Assoc 1997;128(7):843–54.
6. Greenwood M, Meechan JG. General medicine and surgery for dental practitioners: part 3. Management of specific medical emergencies in dental practice. Br Dent J 2014;217(1):21–6.
7. Kufta K, Saraghi M, Giannakopoulos H. Cardiovascular considerations for the dental practitioner. 2. Management of cardiac emergencies. Gen Dent 2018;66(1):49–53.
8. Miller TH, Kruse JE. Evaluation of syncope. Am Fam Physician 2005;72(8):1492–500.
9. Gauer RL. Evaluation of syncope. Am Fam Physician 2011;84(6):640–50.
10. Pallais JC, Schlozman SC, Puig A, et al. Fainting, swooning, and syncope. Prim Care Companion CNS Disord 2011;13(4). https://doi.org/10.4088/PCC.11f01187.
11. Grossman SA, Badireddy M. Syncope. 2022. In: StatPearls [Internet]. StatPearls Publishing. Treasure Island (FL) 2023.

A Patient with a History of Myocardial Infarction and a Stent Presenting for Full Mouth Extractions

Nikhil Mistry, DMD, MD[a], Kenneth Kufta, DMD, MD[a],
Mel Mupparapu, DMD, MDS[b],*, Neeraj Panchal, DMD, MD, MA[c]

KEYWORDS

- Cardiopulmonary arrest • Hypertension • Hyperlipidemia • Myocardial infarction
- Coronary artery disease

KEY POINTS

- In a patient with a history of myocardial infarction and a prior stent placement, acute chest pain in the dental chair could potentially be a cardiopulmonary arrest, which is characterized by a cessation of adequate heart function and respiration that can result in serious morbidity and even death. This scenario primarily focuses on cardiopulmonary arrest.
- Immediate recognition of signs and symptoms of cardiopulmonary arrest is crucial in providing the best chance for optimizing patient outcomes.
- Patients may require surgical, pharmacologic, and radiologic interventions to improve future outcomes. Patients may also be candidates for implantable cardioverter-defibrillators, depending on the nature of their illness.

MEDICAL SCENARIO

A 78-year-old patient arrives with his wife to the oral surgery clinic for extraction of his remaining teeth. The patient is going to be receiving an immediate denture following the extractions. His medical history is significant for myocardial infarction 3 years ago, hypertension, hyperlipidemia, type 2 diabetes, and a 60-pack-year smoking history. Surgical history is significant for stent placement in the patient's left anterior descending coronary artery 3 years ago following myocardial infarction. On examination, the patient's vitals were blood pressure, 186/100; pulse, 88; and respiratory rate, 20. While performing an oral examination, the dentist notices the patient massage his

[a] Hospital of the University of Pennsylvania, Philadelphia, PA, USA; [b] Penn Dental Medicine, Philadelphia, PA, USA; [c] Penn Dental Medicine, Penn Presbyterian Medical Center, VA Hospitals, Philadelphia, PA, USA
* Corresponding author.
E-mail address: mmd@upenn.edu

Dent Clin N Am 67 (2023) 503–506
https://doi.org/10.1016/j.cden.2023.02.030
0011-8532/23/© 2023 Elsevier Inc. All rights reserved.

left chest and wince in pain. The patient complains of chest tightness and extreme dizziness. Without warning, the patient loses consciousness, and his arms fall to his side.

DENTAL MANAGEMENT

The dentist should be immediately concerned that the patient is undergoing cardiopulmonary arrest. Cardiopulmonary arrest is characterized by a cessation of adequate heart function and respiration that can result in serious morbidity and even death. There are various causes of cardiopulmonary arrest, with approximately 75% of cardiac arrest incidences due to underlying coronary artery disease.[1] Other causes of cardiopulmonary arrest include hypovolemia, hypoxia, hypothermia, hypokalemia/ hyperkalemia, acidosis, tension pneumothorax, toxic overdose of drugs, thromboembolism/pulmonary embolism, acute myocardial infarction, and cardiac tamponade.[1] Early prodromes of cardiopulmonary arrest are often present, and these symptoms can include dyspnea, chest pain, palpitations, irregular heartbeats, shortness of breath, weakness, faintness, and lightheadedness or dizziness.[1–3] Signs of cardiopulmonary arrest are often immediate and drastic. These signs include pulselessness, apnea, loss of consciousness, and sudden collapse.[1] Immediate recognition of signs and symptoms of cardiopulmonary arrest is crucial in providing the best chance for optimizing patient outcomes.

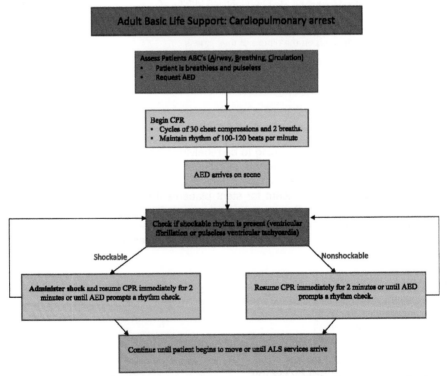

Fig. 1. BLS flow chart.[1,4,9] ALS, advanced life support; CPR, cardiopulmonary resuscitation.

There are 5 key steps in managing a patient with confirmed cardiopulmonary arrest:

1. Confirming cardiopulmonary arrest and beginning basic life support (BLS). **Fig. 1** provides a BLS algorithm.
   - As with any medical emergency, the clinician must assess the patient's ABC's (airway, breathing, and circulation), which will aid in a prompt diagnosis.
   - Once it is determined that the patient is pulseless and/or apneic, proper cardiopulmonary resuscitation must commence immediately.[1,4]
   - As per the clinicians BLS guidelines, chest compressions should be started immediately in a ratio of 30 chest compressions to 2 rescue breaths for an adult and at a rate of 120 compressions per minute.
   - The chest should be compressed at a depth of 2 inches for an adult and should allow for adequate chest recoil.[1,4]
2. Defibrillation: While chest compressions and rescue breaths are ongoing, an automated external defibrillator (AED) should be brought to the scene. Without stopping chest compressions, the AED pads should be placed on the patient's chest, and the pads must be plugged into the device and turned on. Once the device is turned on, chest compressions should continue as the AED begins to analyze the patient's cardiac rhythm. Instructions should be followed as directed by the device to ensure the shock is delivered appropriately. An AED will deliver a shock if ventricular fibrillation or pulseless ventricular tachycardia is detected, with chest compressions briefly stopped during this time. Once the shock is delivered, chest compressions should be immediately resumed.[1]
3. Advanced cardiac life support: This stage is designed to deliver ventilation, stabilize blood pressure and cardiac output, control cardiac arrhythmias, and restore organ perfusion.
   - This is accomplished via defibrillation and cardiac pacing, mechanical ventilation with an advanced airway and intubation, and insertion of an intravenous (IV) line for emergency pharmacotherapy delivery.[1,5]
   - For nonshockable rhythms or after failed defibrillation:
     i. 1 mg of epinephrine should be administered via IV to aid in the return to spontaneous circulation.[6]
     ii. This can be repeated after 3 to 5 minutes.
   - Antiarrhythmic therapy using amiodarone or lidocaine can be started after repeated failed defibrillation and continued electrical instability.
     i. An initial 300 mg IV/intraosseous (IO) bolus of amiodarone or 1 to 1.5 mg/kg IV/IO of lidocaine can be administered.[7]
     ii. A second dose of 150 mg IV/IO of amiodarone can be administered if cardioversion was not achieved.
     iii. Once conversion is achieved, amiodarone 1 mg/h should be given for 6 hours followed by 0.5 mg/h for 18 hours. If lidocaine was used and no conversion was achieved, a second dose of 0.5 to 0.75 mg/kg IV/IO can be administered in 5- to 10-minute intervals.[7]
4. Postresuscitation care: Once successful return to spontaneous circulation is achieved, postresuscitation care should begin. Cardiac arrest can be caused by several diseases and can result in long-term damage to multiple organ systems. Therefore, postresuscitation care focuses on determining and treating the underlying cause of the cardiopulmonary arrest.[8]
5. Long-term management: After survival from cardiopulmonary arrest without irreversible neurologic damage, comprehensive investigation into the nature of the cause is crucial. Patients may require surgical, pharmacologic, and radiologic

Mistry et al

interventions to improve future outcomes. Patients may also be candidates for implantable cardioverter-defibrillators depending on the nature of their illness.[1]

CLINICS CARE POINTS

- Dental treatment in a patient with a history of Myocardial infarction (MI) and a prior stent can be challenging especially if there is a second episode of MI in the chair or waiting room.
- Basic CPR should be perfomed immediately followed by an AED application. An advanced cardian life support can be delivered subject to availability or the patient can be trasferred to a hospital ED.
- The dental treatment can only be resumed if the patient becomes stable and ambulatory.
- It is mandatory to check the patient's medications to make sure that no surgical dental procedure is started without looking into patient's anticoagulation status and patient's use of blood thinners.
- Long-term management of patients who recovered from cardiopulmonary arrest include interdisciplinary team approach where the dentist evaluates the safety aspects of subjecting the patient to a dental procedure in the wake of an MI or even an implanted cardioverter-defibrillator.

DISCLOSURE

The authors have nothing to disclose.

REFERENCES

1. Sharabi AF, Singh A. Cardiopulmonary Arrest In Adults. 2023. In: *StatPearls [Internet]*. FL: StatPearls Publishing, Treasure Island; 2023.
2. Jevon P. Updated posters to help manage medical emergencies in the dental practice. Br Dent J 2015;219(5):227–9.
3. Malamed SF. Emergency medicine: beyond the basics. J Am Dent Assoc 1997;128(7):843–54.
4. Kleinman ME, Brennan EE, Goldberger ZD, et al. Part 5: Adult Basic Life Support and Cardiopulmonary Resuscitation Quality: 2015 American Heart Association Guidelines Update for Cardiopulmonary Resuscitation and Emergency Cardiovascular Care. Circulation 2015;132(18 Suppl 2):S414–35.
5. Merchant RM, Topjian AA, Panchal AR, et al. Part 1: Executive Summary: 2020 American Heart Association Guidelines for Cardiopulmonary Resuscitation and Emergency Cardiovascular Care. Circulation 2020;142(16_suppl_2):S337–57.
6. Long B, Koyfman A. Emergency Medicine Myths: Epinephrine in Cardiac Arrest. J Emerg Med. Jun 2017;52(6):809–14.
7. Panchal AR, Berg KM, Kudenchuk PJ, et al. 2018 American Heart Association Focused Update on Advanced Cardiovascular Life Support Use of Antiarrhythmic Drugs During and Immediately After Cardiac Arrest: An Update to the American Heart Association Guidelines for Cardiopulmonary Resuscitation and Emergency Cardiovascular Care. Circulation 2018;138(23):e740–9.
8. Callaway CW, Donnino MW, Fink EL, et al. Part 8: Post-Cardiac Arrest Care: 2015 American Heart Association Guidelines Update for Cardiopulmonary Resuscitation and Emergency Cardiovascular Care. Circulation 2015;132(18 Suppl 2):S465–82.
9. Alexander RE. A review of changes in the American Heart Association's "Guidelines 2000" for CPR (BLS). Tex Dent J 2000;117(10):73–81.

A Patient with Epilepsy Presenting for a Dental Hygiene Visit

Nikhil Mistry, DMD, MD[a], Kenneth Kufta, DMD, MD[a],
Mel Mupparapu, DMD, MDS[b],*, Neeraj Panchal, DMD, MD, MA[c]

KEYWORDS

- Epilepsy • Photosensitivity • Transient ischemic attack • Seizure • Lorazepam
- Hypotension • Arrythmias • Emergency medical services

KEY POINTS

- Seizures can result from multiple causes, including epilepsy, metabolic abnormalities (alcohol withdrawal, hypoglycemia, hyperglycemia, and electrolyte disturbances), acute brain injury, and reflex epilepsies (photosensitivity or visual sensitivity.
- Seizures may sometimes occur idiopathically, without any known underlying cause.
- Seizures can be classified as being *focal*, in which the neuronal network of one lobe or hemisphere is involved, or *generalized*, in which both hemispheres are involved.

MEDICAL SCENARIO

A 45-year-old woman arrives to the dental clinic for a 6-month periodic evaluation and dental cleaning. Her medical history is significant for several epileptic episodes throughout her life, starting when she was a child. These episodes are usually brought on by staring at flashing lights, and her most recent epileptic episode was 2 years ago. The patient also has a history of hypertension, gastroesophageal reflux disease, and seasonal allergies. Surgical history is significant for appendix removal 10 years ago. On general examination, the patient is alert and oriented and well-appearing. Vitals were within normal limits and well-controlled with the patient's medications. After performing a complete head and neck examination and assessing intraorally, the dentist begins using the Cavitron (Dentsply International, Lancaster, PA 17601, USA) to clean patient's teeth. Suddenly, the clinic loses power, and the emergency light directly above the dental chair starts flashing. The backup generators kick in within 10 seconds, and when the dentist looks down to continue the cleaning, the patient was found

[a] Oral and Maxillofacial Surgeons, Hospital of the University of Pennsylvania, Philadelphia, PA, USA; [b] Penn Dental Medicine, Philadelphia, PA, USA; [c] Penn Dental Medicine, Penn Presbyterian Medical Center, Philadelphia VA Hospitals, Philadelphia, PA, USA
* Corresponding author.
E-mail address: mmd@upenn.edu

rhythmically shaking her extremities, also with notable lip smacking, tongue biting, and moderate frothing foam extruding from the mouth.

DENTAL MANAGEMENT

The dentist should be concerned that this patient with a history of epilepsy is having an acute seizure brought on by the sudden flashing lights. Along with syncope and angina, seizures are one of the most common medical emergencies. Seizures can result from multiple causes, including epilepsy, metabolic abnormalities (ie, alcohol withdrawal, hypoglycemia, hyperglycemia, and electrolyte disturbances), acute brain injury, and reflex epilepsies (photosensitivity or visual sensitivity). Seizures may sometimes occur idiopathically, without any known underlying cause.[1,2] Being able to differentiate the symptoms of an acute seizure from paroxysmal events that can present similarly with migraines, transient ischemic attack, movement disorders, sleep disorders, panic attacks, and even syncope is crucial in providing appropriate management and treatment.[3]

Seizures can be classified as being *focal*, in which the neuronal network of one lobe or hemisphere is involved, or *generalized*, in which both hemispheres are involved.[3] Patients experiencing a focal seizure can have motor (atonic, clonic, spasms, hyperkinetic, myoclonic, and tonic movements) or nonmotor onsets (autonomic, behavior arrest, cognitive, emotional, or sensory deficits) that can be focal at first and can progress to bilateral tonic-clonic seizure. Patients experiencing a generalized seizure can present with abnormal motor movements (tonic-clonic, clonic, tonic, myoclonic, atonic, and spasms) or nonmotor absence seizures.[4] Patients often present with prodromal aura symptoms, during which they experience a subjective experience of a physical or sensory change that is different from normal.[5] This prodrome is then followed by a wide array of possible seizure manifestations, including altered awareness/consciousness, motor manifestations (lip smacking, tongue biting, extremity movements), partial or full-body tonicity phase, and/or partial or full-body clonic movements in which the body moves more rhythmically. These symptoms are often accompanied by frothing at the mouth and urinary incontinence. Other manifestations that are sometimes more difficult to recognize include paresthesia, noisy breathing, olfactory or auditory phenomenon, and déjà vu.[1,6,7] Being able to recognize these clinical symptoms as manifestations of seizure and differentiating them from other emergencies is the first step in proper management.

Once a seizure is suspected and other causes of altered consciousness or involuntary motor movements are ruled out, proper management should commence. The first step in management is to immediately remove/stop all provocative factors (ie, bright flashing lights, drill sounds).[3] The patient should be carefully moved to a flat surface and turned to their side, and all objects that could potentially injure the patient should be moved away.[6] The patients ABC's (airway, breathing, and circulation) should be then assessed and continually evaluated throughout the event, with an intravenous line being placed if possible. Patients with known diabetes mellitus and a new-onset seizure should have their blood glucose levels checked immediately. If blood glucose is less than 60 mg/dL, 1 mg of glucagon should be given intravenously or intramuscularly.[8,9] Most seizures are self-limiting and will stop within a few minutes without pharmacologic intervention. *Status epilepticus* occurs when the patient continues to seize over a period of 5 minutes without returning to a normal level of consciousness. Emergency medical services should be activated, and drug treatment should typically be initiated when a seizure does not resolve within 3 minutes. Benzodiazepines remain as the first-line therapy for patients with continued seizures.

Clinicians should begin administering 4 mg of lorazepam intravenously every 5 to 10 minutes if the seizure continues, 10 mg of midazolam intravenously or intramuscularly every 5 to 10 minutes if the seizure continues, or 10 mg of diazepam intravenously every 10 minutes if the seizure continues.[1] If intravenous administration is not possible, the clinician can administer 0.2 mg/kg intravenous midazolam intranasally or 0.2 to 0.5 mg/kg diazepam gel rectally.[10,11]

Although diazepam has a faster onset of action, lorazepam should be administered because of its longer duration of action.[12] Clinicians should continue to monitor the patient's vitals, particularly their respiratory rate and oxygen saturation, given the respiratory depressive effects of benzodiazepines, while waiting for arrival of emergency medical services.[1] If benzodiazepine treatment is ineffective, a second-line treatment can be attempted by administering either fosphenytoin, valproate, or levetiracetam. A clinician can intravenously administer 20 mg/kg of fosphenytoin up to 1500 mg, 40 mg/kg of valproate up to 300 mg, or 60 mg/kg of levetiracetam up to 4500 mg.[1,6] The patient's vitals should be monitored continuously for unfavorable medication side effects, such as hypotension or arrythmias.

CLINICS CARE POINTS

- Once seizure is uspected, the first step in the management is to remove all provocative factors ans check the airway, breathing and circulation.
- In diabetic patients, if blood sugar is less than 60 mg/dL, 1 mg of glucagon should be given IM or IV.
- Bennzodiazepines remain as the first-line therapy for continued seizures.
- If Benzodiazepines are not effective, a second-line treatment is the use of either fosphenytoin, valproate, or levetiracetam in appropriate doses.
- The patients vitals should be monitored continuously for possible hypotension or arrythmias.

DISCLOSURE

The authors have nothing to disclose.

REFERENCES

1. Huff JS, Murr N. Seizure, StatPearls, 7. Treasure Island, FL: StatPearls Publishing; 2023.
2. Okudan ZV, Ozkara C. Reflex epilepsy: triggers and management strategies. Neuropsychiatr Dis Treat 2018;14:327–37.
3. Gavvala JR, Schuele SU. New-Onset Seizure in Adults and Adolescents: A Review. JAMA 2016;316(24):2657–68.
4. Fisher RS, Cross JH, D'Souza C, et al. Instruction manual for the ILAE 2017 operational classification of seizure types. Epilepsia 2017;58(4):531–42.
5. Spencer D. Auras Are Frequent in Patients With Generalized Epilepsy. Epilepsy Currr 2015;15(2):75–7.
6. Bank AM, Bazil CW. Emergency Management of Epilepsy and Seizures. Semin Neurol 2019;39(1):73–81.
7. Jevon P. Updated posters to help manage medical emergencies in the dental practice. Br Dent J 2015;219(5):227–9.

8. Villani M, de Courten B, Zoungas S. Emergency treatment of hypoglycaemia: a guideline and evidence review. Diabet Med. Sep 2017;34(9):1205–11.

9. Mathew P, Thoppil D. StatPearls, Hypoglycemia. Treasure Island, FL: StatPearls Publishing; 2022.

10. Leppik IE, Patel SI. Intramuscular and rectal therapies of acute seizures. Epilepsy Behav 2015;49:307–12.

11. Wermeling DP. Intranasal delivery of antiepileptic medications for treatment of seizures. Neurotherapeutics 2009;6(2):352–8.

12. De Waele L, Boon P, Ceulemans B, et al. First line management of prolonged convulsive seizures in children and adults: good practice points. Acta Neurol Belg 2013;113(4):375–80.

Foreign Body Aspiration in an Elderly Male with No Significant Medical History

Nikhil Mistry, DMD, MD[a], Kenneth Kufta, DMD, MD[a],
Mel Mupparapu, DMD, MDS[b],*, Neeraj Panchal, DMD, MD, MA[c]

KEYWORDS

- Aspiration • Foreign body • Stridor • Chocking • Wheezing • Airway

KEY POINTS

- Accidental foreign body aspiration remains a real risk during any dental procedure.
- Risk factors for aspiration include young age (1–3 years old), older age, sedative state, altered level of consciousness, obesity, pregnancy, intoxication, intellectual disability, and inappropriate gag or swallowing reflex.
- Prevention of this medical emergency can be accomplished by the use of throat packs and vigilant suctioning throughout the procedure.
- Assistance with dislodgment of the foreign body can be attempted with abdominal thrusts (Heimlich maneuver) or with repeated back blows.

MEDICAL SCENARIO

A 88-year-old man presents to the dental clinic for placement of his final zirconium crown for tooth #18. Medical history is significant for well-controlled hypertension, type 2 diabetes, and hypothyroidism. Patient has no known drug allergies. The patient's vitals and physical examination are noncontributory. The dentist removes the patient's temporary crown on tooth #18, which was cemented with temporary cement. After cleaning off the remnants of the temporary cement, the dentist places a piece of 4 × 4 gauze in the back of the patient's mouth and then tries in the final zirconia crown to confirm appropriate seating and occlusion before final cementation. Although attempting to remove the final crown, the dentist loses grip and the crown falls behind the 4 × 4 gauze and into the patient's posterior oropharynx.

[a] Hospital of the University of Pennsylvania, Philadelphia, PA, USA; [b] Penn Dental Medicine, Philadelphia, PA, USA; [c] Penn Dental Medicine, Penn Presbyterian Medical Center, Philadelphia VA Hospitals, Philadelphia, PA, USA
* Corresponding author.
E-mail address: mmd@upenn.edu

Dent Clin N Am 67 (2023) 511–514
https://doi.org/10.1016/j.cden.2023.02.032
0011-8532/23/© 2023 Elsevier Inc. All rights reserved.

DENTAL MANAGEMENT

Despite following appropriate precautions during clinical procedures, accidental foreign body aspiration remains a real risk during any dental procedure. Foreign body aspiration is among the most common respiratory emergencies within a dental clinic and is the fourth leading cause of unintentional deaths.[1] Although approximately 50% of patients are asymptomatic after aspiration of a foreign body, understanding the appropriate next steps in management of these patients is critical in preventing morbid and even lethal outcomes.[2] Certain subsets of patients are deemed higher risk for aspiration. Risk factors for aspiration include young age (1–3 years old), older age, sedative state, altered level of consciousness, obesity, pregnancy, intoxication, intellectual disability, and inappropriate gag or swallowing reflex.[3] For clinicians treating patients under sedation, awareness of the effect of sedative medications on protective swallowing and cough reflexes is crucial in preventing and treating foreign body aspiration.[3] Patients who experience foreign body aspiration do not always present with acute symptoms following an event and can by clinically asymptomatic. Those patients who experience symptoms often demonstrate acute dyspnea, cough, stridor, choking, wheezing, respiratory difficulty with and without cyanosis, decrease in oxygen saturation, and even eventual loss of consciousness.[3–5] Long-term effects of aspiration can result in vocal cord paralysis, post-obstructive pneumonia, atelectasis, bronchiectasis, pneumothorax, hemorrhage, lung abscess, and even death.[3,5,6]

Clinicians should be vigilant during all dental-related care to minimize the occurrence of these emergencies and also to quickly identify any aspiration event to appropriately manage the patient to optimize outcomes. Prevention of this medical emergency can be accomplished by the use of throat packs and vigilant suctioning throughout the procedure. However, accidental aspiration can happen even with appropriate preventive measures, primarily in the higher risk populations described above. The first step in treating a suspected foreign body aspiration is to remove all materials from the oral cavity and to determine if the patient has an airway obstruction. The clinician should maintain the patient in a supine or reclined position. If the patient is symptomatic and has signs of an acute airway obstruction, they should be asked to cough in attempt to dislodge any objects within the airway. In addition, the clinician may attempt to remove the object with a finger sweep only if able to visualize the object. If the patient is sedated, the clinician can also use a laryngoscope to visualize the hypopharynx and Magill forceps to remove the object. Assistance with dislodgment of the foreign body can also be attempted with abdominal thrusts (Heimlich maneuver) or with repeated back blows. If the retrieval is not achieved after these brief attempts, emergency medical services should be contacted immediately.[3] If the patient becomes unresponsive during this time, the patient's airway, breathing, and circulation should be assessed, and ccardiopulmonary resuscitation (CPR) initiated if necessary. Although undergoing CPR, the airway should be regularly monitored to identify the appearance of the foreign body in the pharynx. A clinician should never perform a blind finger sweep of the throat because the foreign body can be pushed further downwards into the larynx.[1]

If the patient does not present with signs or symptoms of airway obstruction, the patient may have either ingested or completely aspirated the foreign body. The patient should be escorted to the emergency room at this time to obtain a chest radiograph to rule out aspiration. If the object is present in the respiratory tract, a bronchoscopy with surgical removal of the aspirated body should be performed by the appropriate medical personnel.[3] If the object is present in the gastrointestinal tract, further management from a specialist should be obtained. **Fig. 1** provides an algorithm for stepwise management of a patient who experiences a foreign body aspiration.

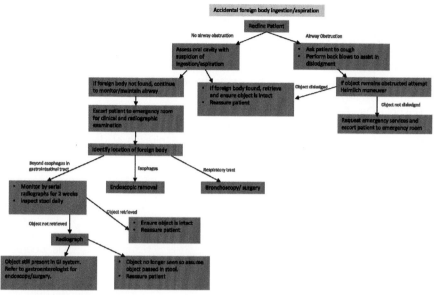

Fig. 1. Flowchart depicting the management of accidental foreign body ingestion or aspiration.[3] GI, gastrointestinal.

CLINICS CARE POINTS

- If an aspiration is suspected in a dental patient, first step is to remove all materials from the oral cavity and instruct the patient to cough to dislodge the foreign body. A finger sweep can be done if the foreign body is visible and should be attempted with the patient in supine or reclined position.

- Abdominal thrusts (Heimlich maneuver) performed or repeated back blows given to dislodge the foreign body.

- If the patient is sedated, a laryngoscope can be used to visualize hypopharynx and a Magill forceps can be used to remove the object.

- A chest radiograph is recommended if there are no signs of distress and if the patient is suspected to have swallowed or completely aspirated. Based on whether the foreign body is in the respiratory track or gastrointestinal tract, appropriate referral is made to a specialist or an emergency department.

- Since this condition is entirely preventable, routine use of throat packs and continuous suctioning and vigilant handling of dental materials is highly recommended.6. Long-term effects of aspiration may lead to vocal cord palsy, pneumonia, atelectasis, bronchiectasis, pneumothorax, hemorrage, lung abscess or even death.

DISCLOSURE

Nothing to disclose.

REFERENCES

1. Dodson H, Cook J. Foreign Body Airway Obstruction. In: StatPearls 6. Treasure Island, FL: StatPearls Publishing; 2023.

2. Doh RM. Foreign body aspiration during dental treatment under general anesthesia: a case report. J Dent Anesth Pain Med 2019;19(2):119–23.
3. Yadav RK, Yadav HK, Chandra A, et al. Accidental aspiration/ingestion of foreign bodies in dentistry: a clinical and legal perspective. Natl J Maxillofac Surg 2015; 6(2):144–51.
4. Limper AH, Prakash UB. Tracheobronchial foreign bodies in adults. Ann Intern Med 1990;112(8):604–9.
5. Basoglu OK, Buduneli N, Cagirici U, et al. Pulmonary aspiration of a two-unit bridge during a deep sleep. J Oral Rehabil 2005;32(6):461–3.
6. Kim E, Noh W, Panchal N. Mortality from an aspiration of dental crown during extraction. Gerodontology 2017;34(4):498–500.

Diabetic Patient in the Chair for Implant Surgery

Nikhil Mistry, DMD, MD[a], Kenneth Kufta, DMD, MD[a], Mel Mupparapu, DMD, MDS[b],*,
Neeraj Panchal, DMD, MD, MA[c]

KEYWORDS

- Insulin • Diabetes mellitus • Hypoglycemia • Hemoglobin A1C • Hypertension
- Hyperlipidemia

KEY POINTS

- Diabetes mellitus is a common medical condition in the United States with 1.5 million new cases diagnosed annually.
- Over a third of adults in the United States have prediabetes, which is characterized as a fasting blood glucose between 100 and 125 mg/dL.
- Hypoglycemia is one of the most dreaded complications among diabetics and remains as one of the leading causes of endocrine medical emergencies.

MEDICAL SCENARIO

A 65-year-old man presents to the dental clinic with his wife for placement of four dental implants to support an overdenture. The patient explained that he rushed to the dental clinic this morning so that he would not be late for his appointment and thus was not able to have much of his morning oatmeal. Medical history is significant for well-controlled type 2 diabetes with daily insulin with meals (Humalog), hyperlipidemia, and hypertension. The patient had an elevated heart rate of 108 beats per minute and a blood pressure of 110/70. Before beginning the procedure, the dentist notices the patient start to sweat and quickly become confused and disoriented while complaining of blurry vision. The dentist retakes the patient's vitals, and the blood pressure has dropped to 98/62 and his heart rate is 125 beats per minute. The patient's hands feel clammy, and his speech was slurred.

[a] Nikhil Mistry and Kenneth Kufa are Oral and Maxillofacial Surgeons at the Hospital of the University of Pennsylvania, Philadelphia, PA, USA; [b] Penn Dental Medicine, Philadelphia, PA, USA; [c] Penn Dental Medicine, Penn Presbyterian Medical Center and Philadelphia VA Hospitals, Philadelphia, PA, USA
* Corresponding author.
E-mail address: mmd@upenn.edu

Dent Clin N Am 67 (2023) 515–517
https://doi.org/10.1016/j.cden.2023.02.033
0011-8532/23/© 2023 Elsevier Inc. All rights reserved.

dental.theclinics.com

DENTAL MANAGEMENT

In a patient with a history of insulin-dependent diabetes in the setting of the signs and symptoms described above, the dentist should be concerned that the patient is experiencing a hypoglycemic episode. Diabetes mellitus affects over 10% of the US population, with over 1.5 million new cases of diabetes diagnosed annually.[1] In addition, over a third of adults in the United States have prediabetes, which is characterized as a fasting blood glucose between 100 and 125 mg/dL or a hemoglobin A1C between 5.7% and 6.4%.[2] Given the tendency of medications used to treat hyperglycemia in diabetic patients to lower blood glucose, patients can present with medication-induced hypoglycemia (defined as <70 mg/dL). Hypoglycemia is one of the most dreaded complications among diabetics and remains as one of the leading causes of endocrine medical emergencies.[3] The signs and symptoms of hypoglycemia do not typically manifest until blood glucose levels are below 55 mg/dL.[4,5] These episodes with dangerously low blood glucose below 55 mg/dL occur in 22% to 34% of type 1 diabetics and 7% to 16.5% of type 2 diabetics. Patients presenting with severe hypoglycemia exhibit a wide array of signs and symptoms, including confusion, dizziness, loss of consciousness, fatigue, nausea, hunger, blurry and double vision, altered speech, convulsions and tremors, anxiety, diaphoresis, and paresthesia.[5]

A clinician's ability to promptly recognize hypoglycemic crises is crucial in preventing serious adverse effects including impaired awareness, reduced quality of life, coma, seizures, and even death.[3] The initial management of this crisis requires assessment of the patient's Airway, Breathing and Circulation (ABCs). The patient's blood glucose should be obtained to confirm a diagnosis of hypoglycemia with a blood glucose below 70 mg/dL. The patient should be placed on 100% oxygen therapy, and all vitals should be continuously monitored. For an alert patient undergoing a hypoglycemic crisis, the patient should be given 15 to 20 g of a readily absorbable carbohydrates such as fruit juice (180 mL), 3 to 4 glucose tablets, or even 15 to 25 mL of sugar—arguably, replenishing with a carbohydrate sources should even be done before measuring blood glucose if there is high suspicion for a hypoglycemic episode.[5,6] Oral glucose or sucrose remains the preferred carbohydrate source for replenishment, as glucose gels and orange juice have been reported to have reduced effectiveness.[3] For patients with altered mental status or for those who are unable to ingest substances by mouth, the patient should be administered 1 mg of glucagon intravenously or intramuscularly.[3,5] Alternatively, 20 to 50 mL of 50% dextrose solution can also be administered intravenously.[6] Once the patient's level of consciousness improves, additional oral glucose can be offered.[7] Another blood glucose sample can be obtained to verify an elevation in the patient's blood glucose levels above 70 mg/dL. Once the patient returns to baseline function with no signs of recurrence, the patient should be monitored for a period of time to determine the need for escalation of care to a hospital setting versus being discharged with instruction to follow up with their primary care physician.[8]

CLINICS CARE POINTS

- Hypoglycemia is one of the most common and dreaded complication among diabetics.
- Patients whose blood sugar is below 55mg/dL may present with dizziness, confusion, loss of consciousness, fatigue, nausea, hunger, blurry or double vision, alteres speech among other symptoms.

- Recommended treatnment depends on the level of consciousness. Alert patients may be given 180 ml of fruit juice, 3-4 tqbs of glucose or 15-25 ml of sugar. In more severe cases, 1 mg of Glucagon can be injected IM or IV or 20-50 ml of 50% Dextrose solution can be administered intravenously (IV). A prompt referral to a hospital for further management is recommended.

DISCLOSURE

Nothing to disclose.

REFERENCES

1. Centers for Disease Control. National Diabetes Statistic Report 2020: Estimates of Diabetes and its burden in the United States. Available at: https://www.cdc.gov/diabetes/pdfs/data/statistics/national-diabetes-statistics-report.pdf. Accessed March 23, 2023.
2. Alvarez S., Coffey R. and Algotar A.M., StatPearls [Internet]. Treasure Island (FL), 2022, StatPearls Publishing, 1–9.
3. Villani M, de Courten B, Zoungas S. Emergency treatment of hypoglycaemia: a guideline and evidence review. Diabet Med 2017;34(9):1205–11.
4. Ford W, Self WH, Slovis C, et al. Diabetes in the Emergency Department and Hospital: Acute Care of Diabetes Patients. Curr Emerg Hosp Med Rep 2013;1(1):1–9.
5. Mathew P, Thoppil D. Hypoglycemia. In: StatPearls [Internet]. Treasure Island (FL). StatPearls Publishing; 2022. p. 1–13.
6. Miller A, Ouanounou A. Diagnosis, Management, and Dental Considerations for the Diabetic Patient. J Can Dent Assoc 2020;86:k8.
7. Jevon P. Updated posters to help manage medical emergencies in the dental practice. Br Dent J 2015;219(5):227–9.
8. Brackenridge A, Wallbank H, Lawrenson RA, et al. Emergency management of diabetes and hypoglycaemia. Emerg Med J 2006;23(3):183–5.

A Patient with an Unknown Latex Allergy Presenting for Sealant Placement

Nikhil Mistry, DMD, MD[a], Mel Mupparapu, DMD, MDS[b],*,
Neeraj Panchal, DMD, MD, MA[c]

KEYWORDS

- Hives • Allergic reaction • Airway • Anaphylaxis • Latex • Rubber dam

KEY POINTS

- In the case of an acute presentation of a hivelike rash soon after exposure to a rubber dam containing latex, the provider should be concerned about an undiagnosed latex allergy.
- Severe allergic reaction to latex-based products is possible, although most reactions remain mild.
- The clinician should promptly assess the patient's airway, breathing, and circulation, with continued monitoring to rule out progression to an anaphylactic reaction.

MEDICAL SCENARIO

A 6-year-old girl presents to a pediatric dental clinic with her mother for sealant place-ment on her first permanent molars. Other than prior prophylactic cleanings, this will be her first dental procedure. The patient has had radiographic bitewings taken in the past, which have not demonstrated any active carious lesions. The dentist lowers the dental chair, and the patient excitedly climbs in all by herself. Medical history is noncontributory, and the patient's mother denies any known drug allergies. The vitals and general examination are normal. On examination, the patient excitedly opens her mouth to show the dentist the new teeth that are coming in. The dentist promises the patient a toy from the toy box if she sits still and keeps her mouth open the entire pro-cedure. The patient now eagerly lays her head back and opens her mouth wide. The dentist is using a latex rubber dam to ensure proper isolation for placing the sealants. Upon placement of the rubber dam, the dentist notes the formation of hives around the patient's face that was in direct contact with the latex rubber dam.

[a] Oral and Maxillofacial Surgeon at the Hospital of the University of Pennsylvania, Philadel-phia, PA, USA; [b] Penn Dental Medicine, Philadelphia, PA, USA; [c] Penn Dental Medicine, Penn Presbyterian Medical Center, Philadelphia VA Hospitals, Philadelphia, PA, USA
* Corresponding author.
E-mail address: mmd@upenn.edu

Dent Clin N Am 67 (2023) 519–521
https://doi.org/10.1016/j.cden.2023.02.034
0011-8532/23/© 2023 Elsevier Inc. All rights reserved.

dental.theclinics.com

DENTAL MANAGEMENT

Given the acute presentation of a hivelike rash soon after exposure to a rubber dam containing latex, the provider should be concerned about an undiagnosed latex allergy. Allergic contact dermatitis occurs when the body's immune system, specifically T cells, are primed to recognize and elicit a localized immune response to an innocuous allergen, such as latex in this scenario.[1,2] A patient's immunoglobulin E binds to this innocuous allergen, causing a release of histamine by mast cells, thus producing this immediate reaction.[3] Although most allergic reactions to latex are mild in nature and often include itching, hives, and rashes,[4,5] severe allergic reactions are possible and may even include anaphylaxis. Obtaining a comprehensive medical history for all new patients before any treatment is crucial, including detailed questioning regarding current medications and known allergies.

Regarding this specific patient scenario, the provider should consider the possibility of an allergic reaction to a substance or material. The dentist should immediately remove the suspected causal material, in this case the latex rubber dam, and continue to closely monitor the patient. The dentist should promptly assess the patient's airway, breathing, and circulation (ABC's), with continued monitoring to rule out progression to an anaphylactic reaction. The dentist should then clean the surfaces of the patient with cool water and mild soap on the skin that was in direct contact with the latex dam.[6] If available, a topical steroid cream can be applied to the affected areas, such as triamcinolone 0.1% (Kenalog) or clobetasol 0.05% (Temovate).[6,7] If the reaction extends more than 20% of the total skin area, a systemic steroid, such as oral prednisone, can be administered for 5 to 7 days to prevent rebound dermatitis.[7] The patient can be administered 0.5 to 1 mg/kg daily of oral prednisone for the next 5 to 7 days. The dentist should also consider administration of a second-generation H1 antihistamine such as diphenhydramine (Benadryl).[8] An adult patient can be administered 25 to 50 mg of oral diphenhydramine with a maximum dose of 300 mg/d, whereas a child can be administered 6.25 to 25 mg of oral diphenhydramine with a maximum dose of 37.5 to 150 mg/d[5,9] The patient should be continually monitored, as progression of an allergic reaction from dermatologic manifestations to systemic symptoms, such as loss of consciousness, or airway or circulation compromise, is possible.[10] The patient can be discharged with a prescription for oral diphenhydramine for 3 days owing to continual circulation of histamine in the bloodstream for 3 days after incident. A pediatric patient can take 25 mg 4 times a day for 3 days, whereas an adult can take 50 mg 4 times a day for 3 days.[5] If the patient's ABC's continue to stay intact after treatment and after appropriate monitoring between 2 and 6 hours, the patient should be discharged with clear instructions to report to the emergency department with the development of respiratory symptoms or any acute symptoms indicating anaphylaxis reaction. Although uncommon, delayed hypersensitivity reactions to the original innocuous allergen, such as latex in this scenario, can present between 4 and 48 hours after initial contact.[11] The patient can present with similar manifestations as an immediate hypersensitivity reaction, including erythema, rubor, swelling, papules, and even local or diffuse edema.[11] The patient should also be sent to a dermatologist or allergy specialist for further evaluation of the suspected latex allergy.[6]

CLINICS CARE POINTS

- If an allergic reaction to latex-based product is suspected, after assessing the ABCs, rule out progression to anaphylaxis.

- Topical steroid creams like triamcinolone 0.1% or clobetasol0.05% is administered topically first and if needed oral administration of Prednisolone 0.5-1 mg/Kg daily for 5-7 days.
- Oral Diphenhydramine 25-50 mg with a maximum dose of 300mg/d can be administered if necessary.
- The patient should be discharged with clear instructions to report to emergency department if respiratory or acute symptoms indicative of anaphylaxis should appear.
- The patient should be referred to a dermatologist or allergy specialist for further evaluation of suspected latex allergy.

DISCLOSURE

The authors have nothing to disclose.

REFERENCES

1. Hamilton RG, Adkinson NF Jr. Mechanisms of acute allergic reactions. Artif Organs 1984;8(3):311–7.
2. Vocanson M, Hennino A, Rozieres A, et al. Effector and regulatory mechanisms in allergic contact dermatitis. Allergy 2009;64(12):1699–714.
3. Abbas M, Moussa M, Akel H. Type I Hypersensitivity Reaction. In: *StatPearls*, StatPearls Publishing. Treasure Island (FL) 2022.
4. Rosenberg MB, Phero JC, Giovannitti JA Jr. Management of allergy and anaphylaxis during oral surgery. Oral Maxillofac Surg Clin North Am 2013;25(3): 401–6, vi.
5. Kenneth L, Reed D. Allergy & Anaphylaxis. Inside Dent 2011;7(3).
6. Nguyen K, Kohli A. Latex Allergy. In: StatPearls. StatPearls Publishing. Treasure Island (FL) 2022;11.
7. Usatine RP, Riojas M. Diagnosis and management of contact dermatitis. Am Fam Physician 2010;82(3):249–55.
8. Schaefer P. Acute and Chronic Urticaria: Evaluation and Treatment. Am Fam Physician 2017;95(11):717–24.
9. Sicari V. and Zabbo C.P., Diphenhydramine, In: StatPearls.11, StatPearls Publishing, 2022, Treasure Island; FL.
10. Alvarez-Perea A, Tanno LK, Baeza ML. How to manage anaphylaxis in primary care. Clin Transl Allergy 2017;7:45.
11. Hamann CP, Kick SA. Update: immediate and delayed hypersensitivity to natural rubber latex. Cutis 1993;52(5):307–11.

Penicillin Allergy in a Patient Presenting for Scaling and Root Planing

Nikhil Mistry, DMD, MD[a], Kenneth Kufta, DMD, MD[a],
Mel Mupparapu, DMD, MDS[b],*, Neeraj Panchal, DMD, MD, MA[c]

KEYWORDS

- Panic attack • Allergic reaction • Local anesthetic • Airway • Anaphylaxis
- Penicillin

KEY POINTS

- It is important for a clinician to appropriately distinguish an anaphylactic reaction from a panic attack or even from a syncopal event.
- Symptoms associated with an anaphylactic reaction include difficulty breathing often secondary to bronchospasm, tachypnea, skin changes such as pruritus and erythema, angioedema, tachycardia, hypotension, and even cardiovascular collapse.
- Even after successful treatment of an acute anaphylactic reaction, anaphylactic reactions may recur within 1 to 72 hours after the original reaction and resolution.

MEDICAL SCENARIO

A 22-year-old man presents to the dental clinic for scaling and root planing of the lower right quadrant. The patient has had previous restorations and cleanings in the past without any complications. Medical history is significant for hypothyroidism. Surgical history is significant for aortic valve replacement 3 months prior. The vitals and general examination are noncontributory. Given the patient's recent valve replacement, the patient's cardiac surgeon advised antibiotics prophylaxis before dental procedures. The patient forgot to take his prescribed 2 g of amoxicillin an hour before his procedure, so the dentist provided the patient 2 g of amoxicillin in the office. Within several minutes of taking the medication, the patient began to experience difficulty in breathing.

[a] Hospital of the University of Pennsylvania, Philadelphia, PA, USA; [b] Penn Dental Medicine, Philadelphia, PA, USA; [c] Penn Dental Medicine, Penn Presbyterian Medical Center, Philadelphia VA Hospitals, Philadelphia, PA, USA
* Corresponding author.
E-mail address: mmd@upenn.edu

Dent Clin N Am 67 (2023) 523–526
https://doi.org/10.1016/j.cden.2023.02.035   **dental.theclinics.com**
0011-8532/23/© 2023 Elsevier Inc. All rights reserved.

DENTAL MANAGEMENT

It is pertinent that dental providers can promptly recognize the signs and symptoms of this medical emergency to provide appropriate treatment. An anaphylactic reaction should be assumed, and a clinician needs to take swift action to prevent potential devastating clinical outcomes. It is important for a clinician to appropriately distinguish an anaphylactic reaction from a panic attack or even from a syncopal event. A patient experiencing a panic attack may present with similar signs including tachycardia, hyperventilation, and even an erythematous rash induced by anxiety.[1] The patient however will not present with urticaria, hypotension, dyspnea, or pallor.[1] A patient experiencing a syncopal event will present with pallor, diaphoresis, hypotension, nausea, and bradycardia.[1] However, they will not present with urticaria, dyspnea, or tachycardia.[1] Symptoms associated with an anaphylactic reaction include difficulty breathing often secondary to bronchospasm, tachypnea, skin changes such as pruritus and erythema, angioedema, tachycardia, hypotension, and even cardiovascular collapse.[1] A patient can also have several gastrointestinal symptoms such as nausea, abdominal cramping and pain, and vomiting.[2,3] Please refer to **Table 1** for additional signs and symptoms of anaphylaxis. Given the wide range of potential systemic symptoms involving several organ systems, anaphylaxis is a potentially life-threatening emergency that requires immediate recognition and attention.[3] The case fatality rate of a patient who experienced an anaphylactic reaction is low at around 0.3% in the United States due to the vigilance of practitioners to recognize and treat these reactions as they occur.[4] Systematically approaching any medical emergency is a key to prompt recognition and allows for increasing the changes of optimal patient outcomes. As per basic life support (BLS) protocol for any emergency situation, the dentist should immediately assess the patient's airway, evaluating for signs of a swollen tongue or throat tightness, stridor, and hoarse voice. Next, the patient's breathing should be assessed (ideally with a stethoscope), noting any chest tightness, wheezing, cough, and/or tachypnea.[1,2,5] The patient's circulation is then assessed by checking carotid or radial pulse, along with measuring blood pressure, and noting any symptoms secondary to hypotension including reflex tachycardia and/or pallor.[1] After appropriate recognition and evaluation of airway breathing and circulations (ABCs), a dentist needs to begin immediate medical management within their appropriate score. Administration of epinephrine remains the most important therapy in treating an anaphylactic reaction, and failure to promptly administer epinephrine remains the most common cause of death associated with anaphylaxis.[1] A patient should be given 0.01 mg/kg of 1:1000 concentration of epinephrine intramuscularly with a maximum

Table 1 Clinical characteristics of anaphylaxis[2,3]	
System	**Signs and Symptoms**
Mucocutaneous	Urticaria, angioedema, erythema, pruritus, diaphoresis
Respiratory	Tachypnea, bronchospasm, shortness of breath, wheezing, stridor, cough, upper airway angioedema, respiratory arrest
Cardiovascular	Tachycardia, hypotension, syncope, pallor, cardiac arrest, bradycardia, arrhythmia
Gastrointestinal	Nausea, vomiting, abdominal cramping and pain, diarrhea
Neurologic	Loss of consciousness, dizziness, drowsiness, irritable, altered mental status, fatigue, malaise
Renal	Urinary urgency or incontinence

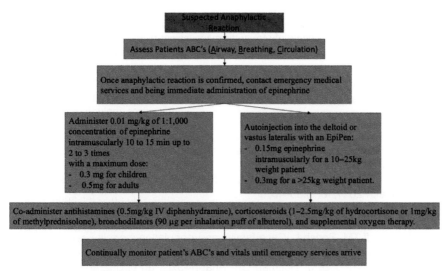

Fig. 1. Schematic representation of anaphylaxis management.[1,3,6,7]

dose of 0.3 mg for children and 0.5 mg for adults every 10 to 15 minutes up to two to three times.[1,6,7] Owing to the detrimental effects of late admiration of epinephrine following a suspected anaphylactic reaction, autoinjectors such as EpiPen were created to aid the medical community in prompt treatment of an anaphylactic reaction. Autoinjection into the deltoid or vastus lateralis with an EpiPen of 0.15 mg epinephrine intramuscularly for a 10 to 25 kg weight patient, or 0.3 mg for a greater than 25 kg weight patient.[3] This dose can be readministered two to three times at 5 to 15 minute intervals if hypotension is still present.[7,8] If intravenous (IV) placement is possible, intravenous administration of epinephrine can also be used for profound broncho-spasm or hypotension. An IV bolus dose of 50 to 200 μg of epinephrine can be administered over 10 minutes followed by 3 minutes of observation for these specific situations.[3] Common adverse effects associated with administration of epinephrine include headaches, anxiety, tremors, dizziness, pallor, and palpitations.[6] Airway patency needs to be assessed continually. The dentist can perform a head tilt and chin lift to open the patient's airway. If unsuccessful, positive pressure ventilation using a bag valve mask or advanced air should be placed.[3] The clinician can also coadminister antihistamines (0.5 mg/kg IV diphenhydramine), corticosteroids (1–2.5 mg/kg of hydrocortisone or 1 mg/kg of methylprednisolone), bronchodilators (90 μg per inhalation puff of albuterol), and supplemental oxygen therapy.[3] Please refer to **Fig. 1** for schematic representation dealing with an anaphylactic emergency. Even after successful treatment of an acute anaphylactic reaction, anaphylactic reactions may recur 1 to 72 hours after original presentation and resolution.[9] A 10 to 24 hour observation period is thus recommended in the event of anaphylactic recurrence.[9]

CLINICS CARE POINTS

- After recognition of the symptoms of anaphylaxis, administration of epinephrine remains the most important therapy for a patient.
- Airway patency needs to be checked continuously in these situations.

- Co-administration of antihistamines, corticosteroids, bronchodilators and supplemental oxygen therapy is the standard of care in the management of anaphylaxis.

DISCLOSURE

Nothing to disclose.

REFERENCES

1. Jevon P, Shamsi S. Management of anaphylaxis in the dental practice: an update. Br Dent J 2020;229(11):721–8.
2. Cheng A. Emergency treatment of anaphylaxis in infants and children. Paediatr Child Health 2011;16(1):35–40.
3. Rosenberg MB, Phero JC, Giovannitti JA Jr. Management of allergy and anaphylaxis during oral surgery. Oral Maxillofac Surg Clin North Am 2013;25(3):401–6, vi.
4. Ma L, Danoff TM, Borish L. Case fatality and population mortality associated with anaphylaxis in the United States. J Allergy Clin Immunol 2014;133(4):1075–83.
5. Maher NG, de Looze J, Hoffman GR. Anaphylaxis: an update for dental practitioners. Aust Dent J 2014;59(2):142–8, quiz 273.
6. Alberto Alvarez-Perea LKT, María L, Baeza ML. How to manage anaphylaxis in primary care. Clin Transl Allergy 2017. https://doi.org/10.1186/s13601-017-0182-7.
7. Tang AW. A practical guide to anaphylaxis. Am Fam Physician 2003;68(7): 1325–32.
8. McLendon K, Sternard BT. Anaphylaxis. StatPearls. StatPearls Publishing; 2023. p. 1–13.
9. Kemp SF. The post-anaphylaxis dilemma: how long is long enough to observe a patient after resolution of symptoms? Curr Allergy Asthma Rep 2008;8(1):45–8.

A Patient with Known Allergy to Local Anesthesia Presenting for a Dental Restoration

Nikhil Mistry, DMD, MD[a], Kenneth Kufta, DMD, MD[a],
Mel Mupparapu, DMD, MDS[b],*, Neeraj Panchal, DMD, MD, MA[c]

KEYWORDS

- Angioedema • Allergic reaction • Local anesthetic • Airway • Epinephrine

KEY POINTS

- Although true allergic reactions to local anesthetic are rare, they should be anticipated especially in a patient with a history of allergies.
- Swollen lips, face, tachycardia, and diaphoresis should warn the dentist to act swiftly for monitoring both cardiovascular and respiratory systems.
- Administration of oral diphenhydramine and continuous monitoring of airway, breathing, and circulation to prevent progression to anaphylaxis is the key to management.

MEDICAL SCENARIO

A 32-year-old woman presents to the dental clinic for an occlusal restoration on tooth #30. The patient has never had any previous restorations and presents to her dentist every 6 months for cleaning and general assessments. Her medical history is significant for asthma, celiac disease, and known allergies to peanuts, latex, and a small rash from local anesthesia from a biopsy of a mole that was performed 15 years ago. The patient is visibly nervous and has a significant fear of needles. On examination, the patient has an elevated heart rate of 112 beats per minute and slightly elevated blood pressure of 146/92. The dentist reclines the patient and talks her through the procedure to help provide a more comfortable environment. The patient's heart rate slows down to 76 beats per minute, and her blood pressure is now 130/88. The dentist applies topical benzocaine to the right cheek. The dentist then performs an inferior alveolar nerve using 1.7 mL of lidocaine with 1:100,000 epinephrine. As the

[a] Hospital of the University of Pennsylvania, Philadelphia, PA, USA; [b] Penn Dental Medicine, Philadelphia, PA, USA; [c] Penn Dental Medicine, Penn Presbyterian Medical Center, Philadelphia VA Hospitals, Philadelphia, PA, USA
* Corresponding author.
E-mail address: mmd@upenn.edu

Dent Clin N Am 67 (2023) 527–529
https://doi.org/10.1016/j.cden.2023.02.036
0011-8532/23/© 2023 Elsevier Inc. All rights reserved.

dentist is waiting for the local anesthetic to take full effect, they notice the patient's lips and lower face begin to swell and that the patient becomes tachycardic and diaphoretic. After a few moments, the dentist notices that the patient begins to develop pruritic hives along her arms, legs, and neck.

DENTAL MANAGEMENT

Although initial signs and symptoms may have signaled dental anxiety/panic attack, the symptoms that develop after administration of the local anesthetic should alert the dentist to consider an acute allergic reaction. Initial signs and symptoms of a panic attack include tachycardia, hyperventilation, and even an erythematous rash induced by anxiety.[1] The patient, however, will not present with facial swelling, lip swelling, urticaria, hypotension, dyspnea, or pallor.[1] The patient has a significant history of allergies and is now experiencing with hives and angioedema-like symptoms after local anesthesia injections. This reaction stresses the important of obtaining a comprehensive medical history, along with performing an in-depth inquiry regarding any reported history of allergic reaction to medications that will be used. The patient is currently presenting with a reaction to the local anesthetic including pruritus and hives. The swollen lips/face, tachycardia, and diaphoresis should be also forewarn the dentist to act swiftly and closely monitor for progression of allergic symptoms that may affect the cardiovascular and respiratory systems.[2]

Management should begin with assessment of the patient's airway, breathing, and circulation (ABCs) per basic life support (BLS) protocol. If ABCs are intact, the dentist should commence with administration of an oral antihistamines. An adult patient can be administered 25 to 50 mg of oral diphenhydramine with a maximum dose of 300 mg/d, whereas a child can be administered 6.25 to 25 mg of oral diphenhydramine with a maximum dose of 37.5 to 150 mg/d.[3,4] After administration of diphenhydramine, the patient's ABCs and vitals should be continuously monitored to exclude progression to an anaphylactic reaction. The next steps in management are dependent on resolution or progression of symptoms. If symptoms do not improve or worsen, emergency medical services (EMS) should be activated and the patient transferred to a hospital as soon as possible. If symptoms resolve on treatment protocols described above, discharging the patient to home can be considered. On discharge, the patient should be given a prescription for oral diphenhydramine for at least 3 days.[3] Clear instructions should be provided to report to the closest emergency department development of symptoms such as wheezing, difficulty breathing, difficulty swallowing, increasing palpitations, and marked intraoral swelling. The patient should also be advised to follow up with an allergy specialist or a dermatologist to perform allergy testing to confirm an allergy to lidocaine or to components of a local anesthetic including preservatives such as bisulfites or methylparaben.[5]

CLINICS CARE POINTS

- Management of any allergic reaction should begin with assessment of patietns airway, breathing and circulation (ABC).
- Diphenhydramine is the first drug fo choice administered orally nopt to exceed a maximum dose of 300mg/d followed by monitoring of ABCs and vitals.
- Patient should be referred to an Emergency Department if the symptoms such as wheezing, difficulty breathing or swallowing, increased palpitations and marked intraoral swelling appear.

- Referral to an allergy specialist or dermatologist is recommended to confirm allergy to local anesthetic including preservatives such as bisulfites or methylparaben.

DISCLOSURE

Nothing to disclose.

REFERENCES

1. Jevon P, Shamsi S. Management of anaphylaxis in the dental practice: an update. Br Dent J 2020;229(11):721–8.
2. Bahar E, Yoon H. Lidocaine: A Local Anesthetic, Its Adverse Effects and Management. Medicina (Kaunas) 2021;57(8). https://doi.org/10.3390/medicina57080782.
3. Joint Task Force on Practice Parameters, American Academy of Allergy, Asthma and Immunology, American College of Allergy, Asthma and Immunology, Joint Council of Allergy, Asthma and Immunology. The diagnosis and management of anaphylaxis: an updated practice parameter. J Allergy Clin Immunol 2005;115(3 Suppl 2):S483–523.
4. Sicari V, Zabbo CP. Diphenhydramine. StatPearls. StatPearls Publishing; 2022. p. 1–9.
5. Arya V, Arora G, Kumar S, et al. Management of patients with allergy to local anesthetics: two case reports. J Dent Anesth Pain Med 2021;21(6):583–7.

Restorative Dental Treatment in a Patient with Mild to Moderate Chronic Kidney Disease (Stages 1–3)

Dalal Alomar, DDS, MS

KEYWORDS

• Restorative • Dental • Treatment • Chronic • Kidney disease

KEY POINTS

- It is important for the dentist to obtain the most recent medical records for CKD patients to reduce the risk of complications and provide the best treatment planning.
- Dentists can proceed with the restorative dental treatment for patients with mildly damaged kidney, CKD stage 2, with no major compilations expected.
- Patients with CKD stage 3 have moderate impairment of renal function with altered drug metabolism, bioavailability, and rate of excretion.
- Pain management for patients with CKD stage 3, include avoidance of NSAIDs and reduction of analgesic drug doses according to the GFR or creatinine clearance.

MEDICAL SCENARIO

A 64-year-old Caucasian man presented to a dental clinic for routine dental examination. Clinical assessment and radiographs revealed carious teeth #12 and #13. The patient's medical history included controlled diabetes mellitus type 2 and chronic kidney disease (CKD). He had stable serum creatinine of 0.9 mg/dL and estimated glomerular filtration rate (eGFR) of 70 mL/min/1.73 m² over the past 6 months, for which he was under conservative treatment. His last hemoglobin A1c was 4.8%. The patient's review of systems and physical examination were negative for abnormal signs and symptoms. The patient was on metformin and vitamin D supplement.

Dental Management Decision and Justification

The patient was considered to have CKD stage 2, with mildly decreased eGFR between 60 and 89 mL/min/1.73 m² according to the National Kidney Foundation classification system for CKD (**Table 1**).[1] In this category of patients, the kidneys are mildly damaged, but still work well. The dentist can proceed with the required restorative

Ministry of Health, Jaber AlAhmad Dental Specialty Center, South Surra, Ministries zone, Kuwait
E-mail address: dalalalomar06@gmail.com

Dent Clin N Am 67 (2023) 531–533
https://doi.org/10.1016/j.cden.2023.02.037
0011-8532/23/© 2023 Elsevier Inc. All rights reserved.

Table 1		
Stages of chronic kidney disease		
Stage	**Description**	**Glomerular Filtration Rate (mL/min/1.73 m²)**
1	Kidney damage with normal or ↑ GFR	≥90
2	Kidney damage with mild ↓ GFR	60–89
3	Moderate ↓ GFR	30–59
4	Severe ↓ GFR	15–29
5	Kidney failure	<15 or dialysis

From National Kidney Foundation. K/DOQI clinical practice guidelines for chronic kidney disease: Evaluation, classification, and stratification. Am J Kidney Dis. 2002;39:S1–266.

dental treatment, which is considered a low-risk non-surgical dental procedure, with no major complications expected. The dentist needs to obtain the most recent medical records including stage of renal disease, systemic comorbidities, recent laboratory tests, risk of bleeding, and medications to reduce the risk of complications and provide the best treatment planning. Blood pressure should be monitored, and stress management protocol should be considered to reduce the risk of stress-related events. Analgesics after restorative dental procedures are not required routinely. The level of renal function for patients with CKD stage 2 is sufficient for the excretion of the drugs and their metabolites with no need for dose adjustment of pain medications.[2] Local anesthetics are metabolized in the liver and generally do not require dose adjustment. Following the medical complexity status (MCS) system, the patient is designated as MSC 1A category.[3]

Patients with CKD stage 3 have moderate impairment of renal function with altered drug metabolism, bioavailability, and rate of excretion. Analgesic management principles should include avoidance of non-steroidal anti-inflammatory drugs (NSAIDs), reduction of analgesic drug doses according to the GFR or creatinine clearance, and close monitoring of drug side effects such as sedation.[4] For pain relief, acetaminophen may be used safely.[5]

Diabetes is a common comorbidity in patients with CKD. In this scenario, the patient is with controlled diabetes and normal hemoglobin A1c level. Please refer to the article on the dental management of patients with diabetes mellitus.

CLINICS CARE POINTS

- Obtain most recent medical records
- Monitor blood pressure
- Consider stress management protocol
- Local anesthetics do not require dose adjustments
- Avoid NSAIDs for patients with CKD stage 3, 4 and 5≈

REFERENCES

1. National Kidney Foundation. K/DOQI clinical practice guidelines for chronic kidney disease: Evaluation, classification, and stratification. Am J Kidney Dis 2002;39: S1–266.

2. Tawfic QA, Bellingham G. Postoperative pain management in patients with chronic kidney disease. J Anaesthesiol Clin Pharmacol 2015;31(1):6–13.
3. Glick M, Greenberg MS, Lockhart PB, et al. Introduction to oral medicine and oral diagnosis: patient evaluation. In: Glick M, Greenberg MS, Lockhart PB, et al, editors. *Burket's oral medicine*. 13th edition. Hoboken, NJ: Wiley-Blackwell; 2021. p. 1–18.
4. Murtagh FE, Chai MO, Donohoe P, et al. The use of opioid analgesia in end-stage renal disease patients managed without dialysis: recommendations for practice. J Pain Palliat Care Pharmacother 2007;21(2):5–16.
5. Munar MY, Singh H. Drug dosing adjustments in patients with chronic kidney disease. Am Fam Physician 2007;75(10):1487–96.

Patient with Severe End-Stage Renal Disease Stages (4–5) Presenting for Surgical Periodontal Therapy

Dalal Alomar, DDS, MS

KEYWORDS

- End-stage renal disease • Periodontitis • Periodontal therapy
- Glomerular filtration rate • Chronic kidney disease

KEY POINTS

- For a patient with severe ESRD, it is important for the dentist to communicate with the patient's nephrologist to obtain the most recent medical records in order to proceed with the surgical periodontal therapy.
- A conservative surgical technique must be followed by the dentist to decrease the risk of bleeding and infection.
- Drug metabolism, bioavailability, and rate of excretion are altered in patients with ESRD, which necessitate adjustments of the dosages and intervals of drugs metabolized by the kidney and avoidance of nephrotoxic drugs.
- Patients with ESRD have an increased risk of bleeding owing to platelet dysfunction associated with uremia.
- Dentists should obtain coagulation tests, follow a conservative surgical technique and ensure the availability of hemostatic agents at the dental office to reduce the risk of bleeding.

MEDICAL SCENARIO

A 67-year-old man was referred from his general dentist for advanced periodontal therapy. He complains of gingival bleeding on brushing, some teeth mobility, and sensitivity. Intraoral examination shows poor oral hygiene, deep gingival pockets, and grade 1 to 2 mobility of posterior teeth. Radiographic examination revealed generalized horizontal bone loss of 2 to 4 mm. The patient had 1 round of nonsurgical periodontal therapy; however, residual deep pockets with subgingival calculus were still present. On the health-history questionnaire, the patient reported that he is hypertensive and was diagnosed with severe end-stage renal disease (ESRD) 1-year ago.

Ministry of Health, Jaber AlAhmad Dental Specialty Center, South Surra, Ministries zone, Kuwait City, Kuwait
E-mail address: dalalalomar06@gmail.com

Dent Clin N Am 67 (2023) 535–538
https://doi.org/10.1016/j.cden.2023.02.038
0011-8532/23/© 2023 Elsevier Inc. All rights reserved.

Table 1
Drug dose adjustments of commonly prescribed drugs in dentistry for patients with chronic kidney disease

Drug Name	Dose	GFR (mL/min)		
		>50	10–50	<10
Analgesics				
Celecoxib (Celebrex)	100–200 mg q12h	Avoid	Avoid	Avoid
Ibuprofen	400–800 mg q8h	Avoid	Avoid	Avoid
Antibiotics				
Amoxicillin	500 mg q8h	No adjustment	q8-12h	q24h
Azithromycin (Zithromax)	250–500 mg q24h	No adjustment	No adjustment	No adjustment
Cephalexin (Keflex)	250–500 mg q6-8h	q8h	q8-12h	q12–24h
Clarithromycin	250–500 mg q12h	No adjustment	50%–100% of usual dose	50% of usual dose
Clindamycin (Cleocin)	150–300 mg q6h	No adjustment	No adjustment	No adjustment
Doxycycline (Vibramycin)	100 mg q12h	No adjustment	No adjustment	No adjustment
Erythromycin	250–500 mg q6h	No adjustment	No adjustment	No adjustment
Metronidazole (Flagyl)	250–500 mg q8-12h	No adjustment	No adjustment	No adjustment
Antifungals				
Fluconazole (Diflucan)	100–200 mg q24h	No adjustment	50% of usual dose	50% of usual dose
Antivirals				
Acyclovir (Zovirax)	200–800 mg q4h	No adjustment	q8h	200 mg q12h

Recommendations for drug use and drug dosing adjustments of commonly prescribed medications in dentistry for patients with chronic kidney disease.

The patient is on losartan, atenolol, hydrochlorothiazide, iron, calcium, and vitamin D supplements. His vital signs were within normal limits. His most recent estimated glomerular filtration rate value was 24 mL/min/1.73 m².

DENTAL MANAGEMENT DECISION AND JUSTIFICATION

For a patient with severe ESRD to proceed with surgical periodontal therapy, it is important for the dentist to communicate with the patient's nephrologist to obtain the most recent medical records, including stage of renal disease, systemic comorbidities, recent laboratory tests, risk of bleeding, and medications to reduce the risk of complications and to provide the best treatment planning. To proceed with periodontal flap debridement, a conservative flap management technique must be followed to reduce risk of complications. Stress management protocol, including a morning appointment and a quiet, calm environment, should be taken into consideration to reduce the risk for stress-related events. Blood pressure should be closely monitored before and during the procedure, and epinephrine-containing anesthetics should be used with caution. Refer toMiriam R. Robbins and Kimberly A. Strauch's article, "Crown Preparation in a Patient with Hypertension and Type 2 Diabetes Mellitus," in this issue for further details on the dental management of hypertensive patients.

Drug metabolism, bioavailability, and rate of excretion are altered in patients with impaired renal function. For this reason, adjustments of the dosages and intervals of drugs metabolized by the kidney must be considered (**Table 1**).[1] Nephrotoxic drugs, such as acyclovir, aminoglycosides, aspirin, non-steroidal anti-inflammatory drugs, and tetracycline, should generally be avoided.[2] Local anesthetics are metabolized in the liver and generally do not require dose adjustment. For postoperative pain management, acetaminophen is generally recommended because it does not cause bleeding and is tolerated better (every 6 hours if glomerular filtration rate [GFR] is 10–50 mL/min and every 8 hours if GFR <10 mL/min).[3] Because of the anemia commonly seen in patients with renal disease, narcotics should be used with caution owing to their respiratory depressant effects.[4]

Patients with ESRD have an increased risk of bleeding owing to platelet dysfunction associated with uremia. It is important to obtain coagulation tests and complete blood count before the surgical procedure, and abnormal values should be discussed with the patient's physician. A conservative surgical technique must be followed to decrease the risk of bleeding and infection. The dentist should ensure the availability of local hemostatic agents at the dental office to be used as needed to obtain hemostasis. Following the medical complexity status (MCS) system, the patient can be designated as MCS 2B category.[5]

CLINICS CARE POINTS

- Obtain most recent medical records.
- Monitor blood pressure before and during the procedure.
- Consider stress management protocol.
- Follow conservative surgical technique.
- Consider djustments of the dosages and intervals of drugs metabolized by the kidney.
- Avoid nephrotoxic drugs.
- Ensure the availability of local hemostatic agents at the dental office.

DISCLOSURE

Nothing to disclose.

REFERENCES

1. Munar MY, Singh H. Drug dosing adjustments in patients with chronic kidney disease. Am Fam Physician 2007;75(10):1487–96.
2. Little JW, Miller CS, Rhodus NL. Chronic kidney disease and dialysis. Little and Falace's dental management of the medically compromised patient. 9th edition. St Louis (MO): Elsevier; 2018. p. 192–209.
3. Brockmann W, Badr M. Chronic kidney disease: pharmacological considerations for the dentist. J Am Dent Assoc 2010 Nov;141(11):1330–9.
4. De Rossi SS, Glick M. Dental considerations for the patient with renal disease receiving hemodialysis. J Am Dent Assoc 1996 Feb;127(2):211–9.
5. Glick M, Greenberg MS, Lockhart PB, et al. Introduction to oral medicine and oral diagnosis: patient evaluation. In: Glick M, Greenberg MS, Lockhart PB, et al, editors. *Burket's oral medicine*. 13th edition. Hoboken, NJ: Wiley-Blackwell; 2021. p. 1–18.

Patient on Hemodialysis Develops Painful Periodontal Abscess and Presents for Treatment

Dalal Alomar, DDS, MS

KEYWORDS

- End-stage renal disease • Hemodialysis • Periodontal abscess • Oral infection

KEY POINTS

- For hemodialysis patients, the arteriovenous shunt arm should not be used for measuring blood pressure or administration of medication.
- The dental procedure should be provided on the day after hemodialysis to reduce the risk of excessive bleeding, as patients are heparinized.
- Dose adjustment may be necessary for drugs that are cleared during hemodialysis where a supplemental dose is given after dialysis.
- The risk of infection of the arteriovenous fistula in hemodialysis patients resulting in septicemia and infective endocarditis is considered low following dental procedures.
- The dentist must follow standard precautions for infection control when treating dialysis patients because the dialysis machine is disinfected, not sterilized.

MEDICAL SCENARIO

A 72-year-old man presented to the dental clinic complaining of painful gingival swelling and bleeding of the right lower quadrant. Periodontal probing revealed accumulation of calculus and abscess within deep ≥6-mm periodontal pockets of vital lower right molar teeth. A panoramic radiograph showed generalized alveolar bone resorption with angular defects of lower right molars. His medical history included end-stage renal disease on dialysis, hypertension, and diabetes mellitus type II. He has been on hemodialysis 3 times per week for the past 2 years with an arteriovenous fistula in the right arm. The patient is on lisinopril, metoprolol, insulin, torsemide, vitamin D, vitamin B12, and iron.

Ministry of Health, Jaber AlAhmad Dental Specialty Center, South Surra, Ministries zone, Kuwait City, Kuwait
E-mail address: dalalalomar06@gmail.com

Dent Clin N Am 67 (2023) 539–541
https://doi.org/10.1016/j.cden.2023.02.039
0011-8532/23/© 2023 Elsevier Inc. All rights reserved.

DENTAL MANAGEMENT DECISION AND JUSTIFICATION

Periodontal abscess is a dental emergency requiring immediate intervention with drainage and mechanical debridement owing to the associated pain and risk of spread of infection. The dentist should obtain most recent medical records, including type of dialysis, degree of kidney dysfunction, systemic comorbidities, recent laboratory tests including coagulation tests, and medications, to reduce the risk of complications and provide the best treatment planning.

Blood pressure should be closely monitored before and during the procedure, and epinephrine-containing anesthetics must be used with caution. Stress management protocol should be considered to reduce the risk for stress-related events. The arteriovenous shunt arm should not be used for measuring blood pressure or administration of medication. The dentist should obtain the level of diabetes control and ensure that the patient has taken his insulin dosage as usual and has eaten his regular meal before the appointment to prevent insulin shock during the dental visit. In patients with poorly controlled diabetes, antibiotics may be prescribed to manage acute dental infections. Refer to the Miriam R. Robbins and Kimberly A. Strauch's article, "Crown Preparation in a Patient with Hypertension and Type 2 Diabetes Mellitus," in this issue.

The dental procedure should be provided on the day after hemodialysis to reduce the risk of excessive bleeding, as patients are heparinized, and the effect of heparin usually lasts for 3 to 6 hours after infusion. If dental care is necessary the day of hemodialysis, consider administering heparin antagonist protamine sulfate (usually by a physician).[1] Local hemostatic agents should be available at the dental office to be used as needed.

Drug metabolism, bioavailability, and rate of excretion are altered in patients with impaired renal function. For this reason, adjustments of the dosages and intervals of drugs metabolized by the kidney must be considered. Nephrotoxic drugs, such as acyclovir, aminoglycosides, aspirin, nonsteroidal anti-inflammatory drugs, and tetracycline, should generally be avoided.[1] For pain relief, acetaminophen may be used safely.[2] Because of the anemia commonly seen in patients with renal disease, narcotics should be used with caution owing to their respiratory depressant effects.[3] Dose adjustment may be necessary for drugs that are cleared during hemodialysis where a supplemental dose is given after dialysis. These drugs include antibiotics, such as amoxicillin and cephalexin. Clindamycin and benzodiazepines are not affected by hemodialysis and may be prescribed at their usual dose without modification.[4] Local anesthetics are metabolized in the liver and generally do not require dose adjustment.

The risk of infection of the arteriovenous fistula (endarteritis) in hemodialysis patients resulting in septicemia and infective endocarditis is considered low following dental procedures. According to the 2021 American Heart Association guidelines on the prevention of infective endocarditis, antibiotic prophylaxis is not indicated for patients with peripheral vascular access used for hemodialysis.

Dialysis patients have an increased risk of acquiring hepatitis B, hepatitis C, and HIV because the dialysis machine is disinfected, not sterilized. Therefore, the dentist must follow standard precautions for infection control when treating dialysis patients. Following the medical complexity status (MCS) system, the patient can be designated as MCS 2B category.[5]

DISCLOSURE

The author has nothing to disclose.

CLINICS CARE POINTS

- Obtain most recent medical records.
- Monitor blood pressure before and during procedure.
- Consider stress management protocol.
- The arteriovenous shunt arm should not be used for measuring blood pressure or administration of medication.
- Provide dental treatment on the day after hemodialysis.
- Avoid nephrotoxic drugs.
- A supplemental dose may be necessary for drugs that are cleared during hemodialysis.
- Follow standard precautions for infection control.

REFERENCES

1. Little JW, Miller CS, Rhodus NL. Chronic kidney disease and dialysis. Little and falace's dental management of the medically compromised patient. 9th edition. St Louis (MO): Elsevier; 2018. p. 192–209.
2. Munar MY, Singh H. Drug dosing adjustments in patients with chronic kidney disease. Am Fam Physician 2007;75(10):1487–96.
3. De Rossi SS, Glick M. Dental considerations for the patient with renal disease receiving hemodialysis. J Am Dent Assoc 1996;127(2):211–9.
4. Kerr AR. Update on renal disease for the dental practitioner. Oral Surg Oral Med Oral Pathol Oral Radiol Endod 2001;92(1):9–16.
5. Glick M, Greenberg MS, Lockhart PB, et al. Introduction to oral medicine and oral diagnosis: patient evaluation. In: Glick M, Greenberg MS, Lockhart PB, et al, editors. *Burket's oral medicine*. 13th edition. Hoboken, NJ: Wiley-Blackwell; 2021. p. 1–18.

Patient on Hemodialysis with Elevated International Normalized Ratio Presents for Removal of Residual Roots in the Mandible

Anwar A. AlMuzaini, DDS, MS

KEYWORDS

● End-stage renal disease ● Hemodialysis ● INR ● Dental extraction ● Oral surgery

KEY POINTS

● Dentists should consult with the patient's physician to obtain the most recent medical records to assess kidney function and disease progression before dental care.
● Dental procedures should be performed the day after hemodialysis to minimize bleeding.
● For patients on anticoagulants, international normalized ratio (INR) should ideally be measured on the day of the procedure. Minor oral surgery can generally be performed if the INR is ≤ 3.5.
● Nephrotoxic drugs should be avoided, and certain drugs may require dose adjustments depending on the patient's glomerular filtration rate.

MEDICAL SCENARIO

A 65-year-old male patient presented for extraction of residual roots of tooth 19. He complained of pain when eating, and the tooth is tender to palpation. Radiographic examination reveals a well-circumscribed radiolucency surrounding the roots. He is diabetic and hypertensive and had been diagnosed with end-stage renal disease (ESRD) and atrial fibrillation 3 years ago. He started hemodialysis shortly after his diagnosis and attends 3 sessions a week. He is currently taking heparin, warfarin, lisinopril, pioglitazone, erythropoietin, iron, vitamin D, vitamin B complex, and folic acid. His most recent international normalized ratio (INR) value, taken 3 days ago, was 3.5.

DENTAL MANAGEMENT DECISION AND JUSTIFICATION

Dentists should obtain the most recent medical records, including a complete blood count, coagulation profile, and renal function tests with glomerular filtration rate

Ministry of Health, 5 Saud Bin Abdulaziz Street, Opposite Public Library, 13022, Kuwait City, Kuwait
E-mail address: a_almuzaini@outlook.com

Dent Clin N Am 67 (2023) 543–545
https://doi.org/10.1016/j.cden.2023.02.040
0011-8532/23/© 2023 Elsevier Inc. All rights reserved.

dental.theclinics.com

(GFR), serum creatinine, and blood urea nitrogen to assess disease progression and medical management. Diabetic control and hypertensive control are also assessed before treatment. Measuring blood pressure is performed on the arm without vascular access.[1] According to the 2021 American Heart Association guidelines on the prevention of infective endocarditis, antibiotic prophylaxis is not indicated for patients with peripheral vascular access used for hemodialysis.[2] Dental treatment should ideally occur the day after dialysis to minimize bleeding.[3] Bleeding may occur, as patients may be anemic, platelet aggregation is impaired, and patients are prescribed anticoagulants to prevent thrombosis of their vascular access.[1] Patients taking warfarin should ideally have their INR measured on the day of the dental procedure or otherwise within 24 hours if it has been stable. The optimal therapeutic INR range will depend on its indication. It is generally safe to perform minor oral surgery (ie, simple tooth extraction) with good local hemostatic measures if the INR is ≤3.5. For higher INR values, a physician consultation is necessary.[4] As renal function is impaired in patients with ESRD, drugs with renal clearance may accumulate, resulting in higher than normal blood levels, and this will necessitate dosage reduction of some drugs (**Table 1**).[3,5] For pain relief, acetaminophen may be used safely.[5] Drugs inherently

Table 1
Drug dose adjustments of commonly prescribed drugs in dentistry for patients with chronic kidney disease

Drug Name	Dose	GFR (mL/min) >50	GFR (mL/min) 10–50	GFR (mL/min) <10
Analgesics				
Celecoxib (Celebrex)	100–200 mg q12h	Avoid	Avoid	Avoid
Ibuprofen	400–800 mg q8h	Avoid	Avoid	Avoid
Antibiotics				
Amoxicillin	500 mg q8h	No adjustment	q8-12h	q24h
Azithromycin (Zithromax)	250–500 mg q24h	No adjustment	No adjustment	No adjustment
Cephalexin (Keflex)	250–500 mg q6-8h	q8h	q8-12h	q12-24h
Clarithromycin	250–500 mg q12h	No adjustment	50%–100% of usual dose	50% of usual dose
Clindamycin (Cleocin)	150–300 mg q6h	No adjustment	No adjustment	No adjustment
Doxycycline (Vibramycin)	100 mg q12h	No adjustment	No adjustment	No adjustment
Erythromycin	250–500 mg q6h	No adjustment	No adjustment	No adjustment
Metronidazole (Flagyl)	250–500 mg q8-12h	No adjustment	No adjustment	No adjustment
Antifungals				
Fluconazole (Diflucan)	100–200 mg q24h	No adjustment	50% of usual dose	50% of usual dose
Antivirals				
Acyclovir (Zovirax)	200–800 mg q4h	No adjustment	q8h	200 mg q12h

Recommendations for drug use and drug dosing adjustments of commonly prescribed medications in dentistry for patients with chronic kidney disease.

nephrotoxic, such as nonsteroidal anti-inflammatory drugs, should be avoided. Dose adjustment may be necessary for drugs that are cleared during hemodialysis where a supplemental dose is given after dialysis. These drugs include antibiotics, such as amoxicillin and cephalexin. Clindamycin and benzodiazepines are not affected by hemodialysis and may be prescribed at their usual dose without modification.[1]

CLINICS CARE POINTS

- Obtain a complete blood count, coagulation profile, and renal function test prior to dental treatment.
- Defer oral surgical treatment if the INR is ≥3.5 and obtain a physician consult.
- Prescribe acetaminophen for pain control
- Avoid NSAIDs.
- Prescribe antibiotics with dose adjustments according to the patient's GFR.

DISCLOSURE

Nothing to disclose.

REFERENCES

1. Kerr AR. Update on renal disease for the dental practitioner. Oral Surg Oral Med Oral Pathol Oral Radiol Endod 2001;92(1):9–16.
2. Wilson WR, Gewitz M, Lockhart PB, et al. Prevention of Viridans Group Streptococcal Infective Endocarditis: A Scientific Statement From the American Heart Association. Circulation 2021;143(20):e963–78.
3. Proctor R, Kumar N, Steain A, et al. Oral and dental aspects of chronic renal failure. J Dent Res 2005;84(3):199–208.
4. Lockhart PB, Gibson J, Pond SH, et al. Dental management considerations for the patient with an acquired coagulopathy. Part 2: Coagulopathies from drugs. Br Dent J 2003;195(9):495–501.
5. Munar MY, Singh H. Drug dosing adjustments in patients with chronic kidney disease. Am Fam Physician 2007;75(10):1487–96.

A Patient with Active Hepatitis B Presents for Dental Extraction

Fatmah Alhendi, BMedSc, DDS, MSOB

KEYWORDS

• Odontology • Management • Hepatitis B • Drugs • Infections • Bleeding

KEY POINTS

- All elective dental treatments for patients with active hepatitis B should be deferred until recovery.
- Urgent dental work should be carried out in an isolated operation room with adherence to the universal standard precautions.
- All health care workers with clinical exposure should be fully vaccinated against hepatitis B.
- Complete blood count, liver function test, and preoperative coagulation profile should be requested, and any abnormalities should be discussed with the patient's physician.
- Medications metabolized by the liver should be avoided.

MEDICAL SCENARIO

A 35-year-old man presented to the clinic for extraction of a painful unrestorable lower molar tooth. Upon history taking, the patient reported being diagnosed with active hepatitis B.

DENTAL MANAGEMENT DECISION AND JUSTIFICATION

For patients who have active hepatitis B, all elective dental treatments should be deferred until recovery, and urgent dental work, as in this case, should be carried out in an isolated operation room with adherence to the standard precautions recommended by the Centers of Disease Control and Prevention and the American Dental Association to prevent cross-infection in the dental practice.[1] In addition, all health care workers with clinical exposure should be fully vaccinated against hepatitis B. [1] In this case scenario, where extraction is required, complete blood count, liver function test, and preoperative coagulation profile, mainly prothrombin time (PT), bleeding time, and international normalized ratio (INR), should be requested, and any

Ministry of health, AlSulaibikhat, Jamal Abdulnasser Street, Kuwait city, Kuwait
E-mail address: fatmaj_13@hotmail.com

Dent Clin N Am 67 (2023) 547–548
https://doi.org/10.1016/j.cden.2023.02.041
0011-8532/23/© 2023 Elsevier Inc. All rights reserved.

abnormalities should be discussed with the patient's physician.[2] Test results confirmed that PT was 13 seconds per control (normal values, 11–13.5 seconds), INR was 2.5 (normal values, 0.8–1.1), platelet count was 160,000/dL (normal values, 150,000–450,000/dL). These laboratory test results suggest that only local measures to control bleeding would be necessary (refer to case no. 40). Medications that are metabolized by the liver, such as some analgesics and antibiotics, should be avoided.[3] Antibiotic prophylaxis is not recommended, but the need of antibiotics depends on the severity of the liver disease and the dental infection.[2] Local anesthesia can be achieved safely with no more than 2 carpules of lidocaine 2% with epinephrine (1:100,000).[2] In this case, the patient was managed under local anesthesia with 1 carpule of lidocaine 2% with epinephrine (1:100,000) for the dental extraction with implementation of local measures to control bleeding, such as tranexamic acid mouth rinse during the first 2 days postoperatively. The patient did not exhibit any signs and symptoms of systemic infection, so antibiotics were not prescribed. The patient was prescribed 2 gm/day of acetaminophen to control pain postoperatively. The aim of dental management of patients with active hepatitis B infection is to defer elective dental treatment as possible, to gain consultation from the patient's physician, and to limit care for pain control, limit treatment of acute infection, and control bleeding until the patient's condition is stabilized.[2] If an oral surgical procedure is required, minimize soft tissue trauma and consider treating the patient in a hospital setting in the case of advanced surgical procedures or abnormal coagulation profile.[2]

CLINICS CARE POINTS

- In patients with active hepatitis B infection, dental treatments are mainly in cases of emergencies to prevent cross infection and other complications associated with liver disease such as bleeding tendency and drug interactions.
- The adherant to the universal standard precautions and vaccination against Hepatitis B reduce the risk of cross infection among health care workers with clinical exposure to the virus.

FINANCIAL SUPPORT AND SPONSORSHIP

Nil.

CONFLICTS OF INTEREST

There are no conflicts of interest.

REFERENCES

1. Kohn WG, Collins AS, Cleveland JL, et al. Guidelines for infection control in dental health-care settings–2003. MMWR Recomm Rep (Morb Mortal Wkly Rep) 2003; 52(Rr-17):1–61.
2. Golla K, Epstein JB, Cabay RJ. Liver disease: current perspectives on medical and dental management. Oral Surg Oral Med Oral Pathol Oral Radiol Endod 2004; 98(5):516–21.
3. Dart RC. The use and effect of analgesics in patients who regularly drink alcohol. Am J Manag Care 2001;7(19 Suppl):S597–601.

A Patient with Alcoholic Liver Disease Reports for Treatment of Dentoalveolar Abscess in Relation to Maxillary Left Molar

Fatmah Alhendi, BMedSc, DDS, MSOB

KEYWORDS

• Alcoholic liver disease • Odontology • Drugs • Infections • Bleeding • Cirrhosis
• Management

KEY POINTS

• Patients with alcoholic liver disease are more prone to postoperative bleeding, depending on the severity of the liver disease.
• Caution must be taken when prescribing medications for patients with alcoholic liver disease, as they may have abnormal drug metabolism.
• Patients with chronic liver disease with comorbidities are more prone to infections, and prophylactic antibiotics may be necessary before surgical procedures.

MEDICAL SCENARIO

A 51-year-old white man presented to the dental clinic with a swelling in relation to the upper-left molar tooth. The clinical and radiographic intraoral examination revealed a dentoalveolar abscess in relation to a carious maxillary left molar. A detailed medical history was taken. The patient has a diagnosis of alcoholic liver disease (ALD) and currently is on naltrexone and disulfiram treatments.

DENTAL MANAGEMENT DECISION AND JUSTIFICATION

Dental management of patients with ALD depends on the understanding of the potential complications associated with the systemic effects of the liver disease on the patient. A comprehensive medical history should be obtained, and the anesthetic and surgical risk of the patient with ALD can be determined using the Child-Pugh classification.[1] Several factors must be evaluated in this classification, including the presence

Ministry of health, Al Sulaibikhat, Jamal Abdulnasser Street, P.O. Box:5, Kuwait city, Kuwait
E-mail address: falhendi@alumni.upenn.edu

Dent Clin N Am 67 (2023) 549–552
https://doi.org/10.1016/j.cden.2023.02.042
0011-8532/23/© 2023 Elsevier Inc. All rights reserved.

or absence of ascites, nutritional status, the presence of encephalopathy, and the levels of serum albumin and bilirubin.[1] In addition, the modified Child-Pugh score (MCP) was found to be associated with increased postoperative bleeding in patients with advanced liver disease undergoing invasive dental procedures[1]: those procedures that can induce bleeding, such as scaling and dental extractions. In addition to those factors included in the original Child-Paugh classification, MCP also takes in to account prothrombin time (PT) and international normalized ratio (INR).[1] Patients with grade A = child-Pugh score have well-compensated liver disease; grade B = significant function compromise; and grade C = decompensated disease.[1] Based on the severity score, additional blood products (eg, fresh-frozen plasma, platelets transfusion, Desmopressin) or local measures (eg, suturing, gel foam) will be implemented (**Table 1**).[1] As the patient in this case scenario needs incision and drainage for the abscess, consideration must be given to the possibility of excessive bleeding during and after oral surgical procedure. This occurs because of the long-term effect of alcohol ingestion on the megakaryocyte maturation and the resulting platelet depletion and the inhibition of the release of thromboxane A and B, important factors for platelet aggregation.[1] The result will be an increase in bleeding time. Moreover, because the liver is responsible for the manufacturing of coagulation factors, such as fibrinogen, prothrombin, and factors V, VII, IX, and X, and the storage of vitamin K, these patients may suffer prolonged PT.[1] Given these facts, a complete blood count, liver function test, and coagulation profile were requested. Test results confirmed that PT was 13 seconds per control (normal value, 11–13.5 seconds), INR was 1.5 (normal value, 1.1 or below), platelet count was 150,000/dL (normal value, 150,000 to 450,000 platelets per microliter of blood), Total serum bilirubin was 1.5 mg/dL (normal value, 0.1 to 1.2 mg/dL), and serum albumin was 3 g/dL (normal value, 3.4 to 5.4 g/dL). No clinical signs of ascites or encephalopathy were noted. The patient is considered grade A (well-compensated disease), and only local measures to control bleeding after incision and drainage were implemented. It is worth noting that patients with ALD may have increased or decreased rate of drug metabolism, including local anesthetics, analgesics, and some antibiotics, depending on the level of hepatocyte destruction[2] (see **Table 1**). In a well-compensated disease, local anesthesia is safe for patients with liver disease. When sedation is required, conscious sedation with nitrous oxide/oxygen is preferable to intravenous sedation with benzodiazepines to avoid oversedation.[2] Clinicians should also be aware of the effect of ALD on the metabolism of medications used to treat dental conditions, as some of these medications are metabolized in the liver. Nonsteroidal anti-inflammatory medications and aspirin may enhance gastric bleeding when taken with alcohol.[2] Long-term alcohol ingestion can result in acetaminophen being converted into a toxic metabolite that can result in severe liver injury, so only low doses of acetaminophen (maximum, 2 g per day) alone or in combination with hydrocodone (Vicodin, Lorcet) or oxycodone (Percocet) are allowed.[2] Also, alcohol inhibits the absorption of the antibiotic, penicillin, so a 3-hour separation between alcohol ingestion and penicillin should be achieved. Moreover, Metronidazole should not be prescribed for patients who ingest alcohol because it can cause disulfiram reaction that can present as headache, nausea, and facial flushing.[3] Patients with ALD are generally treated with naltrexone and disulfiram, as in this case. Patients being treated with naltrexone that require opioid analgesics should discontinue the naltrexone 48 hours before the dental procedure after consultation with the patient's physician, as naltrexone will decrease the analgesic effect of the opioids if coadministered.[4] Patients with advanced liver disease, such as liver cirrhosis, or with comorbidities, such as cardiac defects, drug abuse, and/or chronic renal failure, are at greater risk for bacterial endocarditis. For that reason, prophylactic

Table 1
Dental management of patient with alcoholic liver disease

Dental Considerations	Child-Pugh Grade A	Child-Pugh Grade B	Child-Pugh Grade C
Antibiotics	Not needed in absence of systemic infection	Consult with patient physician if liver cirrhosis with comorbidities for the need of prophylactic antibiotics	Consult with patient physician if liver cirrhosis with comorbidities for the need of prophylactic antibiotics
Hemostatic measures in invasive dental procedures	• *Local hemostatic agents:* Tranexamic acid rinse, epsilon aminocaproic acid rinse • *Local hemostatic measures:* Suturing, gel foam, Oxycel, Surgicel, or microfibrillar collagen	• Local hemostatic agents and measures, fresh-frozen plasma, vitamin K, platelets (if <50,000 μL for low-risk dental procedures, <100,000 μL for high-risk surgical dental procedures with a higher risk of bleeding), antifibrinolytics • If INR >2, platelets <50,000/μL, consult with hematologist to assess administration of Desmopressin in a hospital setting	• Local hemostatic agents and measures, fresh-frozen plasma, vitamin K, platelets (if <50,000 μL for low-risk dental procedures, <100,000 μL for high-risk surgical dental procedures with a higher risk of bleeding), antifibrinolytics • If INR >2, platelets <50,000/μL, consult with hematologist to assess administration of Desmopressin in a hospital setting
Drug metabolism: Local anesthetics, sedative, hypnotic drugs, and general anesthesia	Enzyme induction is likely to occur, larger than normal doses may be required	Enzyme induction or diminishing can occur	Enzyme diminishing less than normal doses or alteration of the medication may be required

administration of 2 g penicillin or 600 mg clindamycin, 1 hour preoperatively may be required if bleeding is expected[5] (see **Table 1**).

In this case, the patient was managed under local anesthesia by lidocaine 2% with epinephrine for incision and drainage with implementation of local measures to control bleeding, such as tranexamic acid mouth rinse during the first 2 days postoperatively. The patient did not exhibit any signs and symptoms of systemic infection and has well-controlled disease (grade A), so antibiotics were not prescribed. The patient was pre-scribed 2 g per day of acetaminophen to control pain and was referred for root canal treatment for the maxillary left molar.

CLINICS CARE POINTS

- To overcome clinical complications in patients with alcoholic liver disease presenting for dental treatment, the severity of the liver disease should be determined.
- Complications of dental treatments in patients with alcoholic liver disease arise from risk of infections, excessive bleeding, and drug interactions.

FINANCIAL SUPPORT AND SPONSORSHIP

Nil.

CONFLICTS OF INTEREST

There are no conflicts of interest.

REFERENCES

1. Valerin MA, Napeñas JJ, Brennan MT, et al. Modified Child-Pugh score as a marker for postoperative bleeding from invasive dental procedures. Oral Surg Oral Med Oral Pathol Oral Radiol Endod 2007;104(1):56–60.
2. Dart RC. The use and effect of analgesics in patients who regularly drink alcohol. Am J Manag Care 2001;7(19 Suppl):S597–601.
3. Williams CS, Woodcock KR. Do ethanol and metronidazole interact to produce a disulfiram-like reaction? Ann Pharmacother 2000;34(2):255–7.
4. Kranzler HR, Modesto-Lowe V, Van Kirk J. Naltrexone vs. nefazodone for treatment of alcohol dependence. A placebo-controlled trial. Neuropsychopharmacology 2000;22(5):493–503.
5. Hung TH, Hsieh YH, Tseng KC, et al. The risk for bacterial endocarditis in cirrhotic patients: a population-based 3-year follow-up study. Int J Infect Dis 2013;17(6): e391–3.

Patient with End-Stage Liver Disease and Prolonged Prothrombin Time Presents for Placement of a New Dental Implant

Anwar A. AlMuzaini, DDS, MS

KEYWORDS

• Cirrhosis • Nonalcoholic fatty liver disease • Dental implant • Oral surgery

KEY POINTS

- Dentists need to consult with the patient's hepatologist to obtain most recent medical records.
- Prolonged prothrombin time is not necessarily an indication of bleeding risk in patients with cirrhosis.
- The Child-Pugh classification for cirrhosis is a better tool to assess risk of infection and bleeding.
- Drug metabolism may be altered and will require dose adjustments of some drugs metabolized by the liver.

MEDICAL SCENARIO

A 55-year-old male patient presents for placement of a dental implant of a nonrestorable maxillary right central incisor. His past medical history is positive for hypertriglyceridemia and low high-density lipoprotein. He has been diagnosed with nonalcoholic fatty liver disease (NAFLD), which recently progressed into NAFLD-induced cirrhosis (or end-stage liver disease). He has been advised by his physician to implement lifestyle modifications relating to diet and exercise. He is currently taking atorvastatin, and he continues to be monitored by his hepatologist for complications. His most recent blood tests (taken 3 months ago) show a prothrombin time (PT) of 22 seconds.

Ministry of Health, 5 Saud Bin Abdulaziz Street, Opposite Public Library, 13022, Kuwait City, Kuwait
E-mail address: a_almuzaini@outlook.com

Dent Clin N Am 67 (2023) 553–555
https://doi.org/10.1016/j.cden.2023.02.043
0011-8532/23/© 2023 Elsevier Inc. All rights reserved.
dental.theclinics.com

Table 1
Recommendations of commonly prescribed drugs in dentistry for patients with cirrhosis

Drug Name	Recommendation
Analgesics	
Acetaminophen	Safe to use in small amounts (<2g/d) for a short duration
NSAIDs	Use cautiously or avoid in advanced cirrhosis
Antibiotics	
Amoxicillin	Safe
Azithromycin	Avoid
Clindamycin	Avoid
Metronidazole	Avoid
Tetracycline	Avoid
Antifungals	
Fluconazole	Use with caution
Miconazole	Use with caution
Antivirals	
Acyclovir	Safe
Valacyclovir	Safe

Drug dose adjustments and recommendations of commonly prescribed drugs in dentistry for patients with cirrhosis.
Data from Lewis, J.H. and J.G. Stine, Review article: prescribing medications in patients with cirrhosis - a practical guide. Aliment Pharmacol Ther, 2013. 37(12): p. 1132-56.

DENTAL MANAGEMENT DECISION AND JUSTIFICATION

Consulting with the hepatologist and obtaining medical records detailing the liver condition and extent of impairment are essential. Complete blood count with differential, coagulation profile and liver function tests should be reviewed before dental treatment.[1] Because of the liver's role in the synthesis of coagulation factors and drug metabolism, bleeding risk and altered drug metabolism are 2 concerns for a patient with cirrhosis undergoing dental treatment.[2] Prolongation of PT in cirrhosis does not necessarily indicate a risk of bleeding, as this can be balanced by a reduced protein C (a liver-derived anticoagulant), which the PT test does not account for. Platelet count and fibrinogen levels are the standard of care in assessing coagulation for patients with cirrhosis.[3] The Child-Pugh classification for cirrhosis is a helpful tool to predict risk of both infection and bleeding.[4] In the absence of other significantly abnormal coagulation or laboratory values, which would necessitate a hepatologist consultation, bleeding may be controlled by minimizing trauma and using local hemostatic measures (eg, applying pressure and using sutures). Drug metabolism may be decreased in the following: elevated aspartate transaminase or alanine aminotransferase greater than 4x, elevated serum bilirubin greater than 2.0 mg/dL, reduced serum albumin less than 3.5 g/dL, and evidence of encephalopathy or ascites due to liver failure; this may necessitate the adjustment or avoidance of certain drugs metabolized in the liver (**Table 1**).[2] Amide local anesthetics metabolized in the liver (eg, lidocaine) are safe to use in an appropriate amount (ie, the minimum dose to achieve local anesthesia).[2] If benzodiazepines have to be used, lorazepam or alprazolam are preferred at low doses and frequency; this is because benzodiazepines may cause or worsen hepatic encephalopathy in patients with cirrhosis.[2] Antibiotic prophylaxis before dental procedures is not currently recommended for patients with cirrhosis.[2]

CLINICS CARE POINTS

- Obtain complete blood count with differential, coagulation profile, and liver function tests prior to dental treatment.
- Do not defer dental treatment in cases with isolated prolonged PT without considering other coagulation parameters.
- Refer to the Child-Pugh classification for cirrhosis to asses risk of infection and bleeding.
- Acetaminophen in small amounts is safe to use for patients with cirrhosis.
- Lidocaine in appropriate amounts is safe to use for local anesthesia.
- Choose lorazepam or alprazolam if benzodiazepine use is necessary.
- Antibiotic prophylaxis is not currently recommended for patients with cirrhosis.

DISCLOSURE

The author has nothing to disclose.

REFERENCES

1. Golla K, Epstein JB, Cabay RJ. Liver disease: current perspectives on medical and dental management. Oral Surg Oral Med Oral Pathol Oral Radiol Endod 2004; 98(5):516–21.
2. Firriolo FJ. Dental management of patients with end-stage liver disease. Dent Clin North Am 2006;50(4):563–90, vii.
3. O'Leary JG, Greenberg CS, Patton HM, et al. AGA clinical practice update: coagulation in cirrhosis. Gastroenterology 2019;157(1):34–43.e1.
4. Lockhart PB, et al. Dental management considerations for the patient with an acquired coagulopathy. Part 1: coagulopathies from systemic disease. Braz Dent J 2003;195(8):439–45.

Patient with Chronic Liver Disease Was Referred for Evaluation of Oral Infection and Facial Swelling and Needs Multiple Dental Extractions

Anwar A. AlMuzaini, DDS, MS

KEYWORDS

- Chronic liver disease • Hepatitis C • Dental extraction • Facial swelling
- Odontogenic infection

KEY POINTS

- Patients with chronic liver disease due to hepatitis C virus may present with a dental emergency necessitating treatment.
- Recent medical records and laboratory values should be obtained. In cases of dental emergencies, this may not be feasible, and contacting the patient's hepatologist is warranted to verify the patient is under good medical management and the condition is stable.
- Implementing standard infection precautions for injection safety and proper sterilization of equipment is important.
- In the absence of severe liver disease. dental extraction can be performed safely in patients with chronic liver disease with minimizing trauma and local hemostatic measures.

MEDICAL SCENARIO

A 60-year-old female patient developed left-sided facial swelling and severe pain 1 day ago. On clinical and radiographic examinations, teeth 18,19, and 20 were grossly cavitated and required extraction. Her last dental visit was 10 years ago, and she has been neglecting her oral health. She has been diagnosed with chronic hepatitis C virus (HCV) 15 years ago and completed subcutaneous pegylated interferon alfa and oral ribavirin without adequate response. She is currently taking ledipasvir/sofosbuvir and shows no signs or symptoms of liver disease. She reports at her last follow-up 1 month ago her hepatologist noted her laboratory values were within normal limits, but she does not have the results.

Ministry of Health, 5 Saud Bin Abdulaziz Street, Opposite Public Library, 13022, Kuwait City, Kuwait
E-mail address: a_almuzaini@outlook.com

Dent Clin N Am 67 (2023) 557–559
https://doi.org/10.1016/j.cden.2023.02.044
0011-8532/23/© 2023 Elsevier Inc. All rights reserved.
dental.theclinics.com

DENTAL MANAGEMENT DECISION AND JUSTIFICATION

As this patient presents with facial swelling due to an odontogenic infection, this constitutes a dental emergency that requires immediate treatment. The source of infection should be identified and extraction performed without delay. In the absence of recent medical records or laboratory values, the dentist may contact the physician and ascertain that the patient's condition is stable and under good medical management. It is important to verify the absence of severe liver dysfunction or presence of active hepatitis before treatment. Patients with active hepatitis should be seen only for urgent care in an isolated operatory with minimization of aerosols.[1] HCV can be transmitted through percutaneous injuries with an approximately 2% risk and can survive for 16 hours on a dry surface; it is important to implement standard precautions for injection safety and proper sterilization of equipment.[2] Although patients with chronic liver disease may have a bleeding tendency, it is not necessary to obtain a coagulation profile (prothrombin time, activated partial-thromboplastin time, or international normalized ratio) before treatment, as they correlate poorly with bleeding in patients with chronic liver disease that has not progressed.[3] To reduce the risk of bleeding, the dentist may extract the offending tooth or teeth only and schedule the extraction of the remaining teeth over multiple visits. Bleeding may be controlled by minimizing trauma and using local hemostatic measures (eg, applying pressure, sutures, or absorbable gelatin sponges). Local anesthetics may be safely administered, as there is no significant liver dysfunction.[4] Commonly prescribed drugs in dentistry that are metabolized by the liver may be used if the patient does not have a history of severe hepatic disease. For antibiotic prescription, the dentist may safely prescribe amoxicillin without dosage adjustment, as it is not mainly metabolized by the liver. Although metronidazole and tetracyclines are metabolized by the liver, they may be prescribed in limited amounts. Postsurgical pain relief for this patient may be achieved with short-term use of acetaminophen or ibuprofen (these are to be avoided in severe liver disease).[1]

CLINICS CARE POINTS

- Verify the absence of severe liver disease or active hepatitis of patients with chronic liver disease prior to dental treatment.
- Do not delay dental extractions in a dental emergency once the necessary records are obtained.
- It is not necessary to obtain a coagulation profile prior to dental treatment for patients with chronic liver disease that has not progressed.
- Amoxicillin is safe to prescribe for patients with chronic liver disease.
- Pain relief is achieved with short-term use of acetaminophen or ibuprofen.

DISCLOSURE

The author has nothing to disclose.

REFERENCES

1. James W, Little CSM, Rhodus NL. Dental management of the medically compromised patient. 9th edition. St. Louis (MO): Elsevier; 2018.

2. Klevens RM, Moorman AC. Hepatitis C virus: an overview for dental health care providers. J Am Dent Assoc 2013;144(12):1340–7.
3. Tripodi A, Mannucci PM. The coagulopathy of chronic liver disease. N Engl J Med 2011;365(2):147–56.
4. Haas DA. An update on local anesthetics in dentistry. J Can Dent Assoc 2002; 68(9):546–51.

Moving?

Make sure your subscription moves with you!

To notify us of your new address, find your **Clinics Account Number** (located on your mailing label above your name), and contact customer service at:

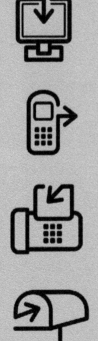

Email: journalscustomerservice-usa@elsevier.com

800-654-2452 (subscribers in the U.S. & Canada)
314-447-8871 (subscribers outside of the U.S. & Canada)

Fax number: 314-447-8029

Elsevier Health Sciences Division
Subscription Customer Service
3251 Riverport Lane
Maryland Heights, MO 63043

*To ensure uninterrupted delivery of your subscription, please notify us at least 4 weeks in advance of move.

Printed and bound by CPI Group (UK) Ltd, Croydon, CR0 4YY

03/10/2024

01040474-0019